I0096479

Medical Logbook:

The Health Care Record Book Designed to Save Your Information and Your Life!

Medical Information

Emergency Contacts

Medical Alerts

Doctor and Medication Information

Health Care Visits

Two Years of Daily Vitals

and MORE!

by

Morgan Williams

Bzik Publishing LLC

Seattle, WA

Copyright ©2025 by Morgan Williams

All rights reserved.

No portion of this book may be reproduced, distributed, or transmitted in any form or by any means, including photocopying, recording, or other electronic or mechanical methods, without the prior written permission of the publisher or author, except in the case of brief quotations embodied in critical reviews and certain other noncommercial uses permitted by U.S. copyright law. For permission requests, write to the author through the publisher at the email below.

All included information is accurate at the time of writing and publishing. You are encouraged to conduct your own research and make the best decisions for yourself based on your personal needs.

Printed and published in the United States of America by Bzik Publishing LLC.

First printing edition 2025.

All inquiries about this book can be sent to the author via publisher.

Email: BzikPublishing@gmail.com

Bzik Publishing LLC

Seattle, WA

Table of Contents

How to Successfully Use This Logbook. 4

General Information 7

Emergency Contacts 8

Medical Alerts for Allergies 8

Medical Conditions Alerts... 8

Doctor Information... 9

Medication Information 10

Medical Visits...11

Personal Vitals Importance...12

Daily Vitals Log: *104 weeks = two full years* 15

Notes...119

How to Successfully Use This Logbook.

This Medical Logbook is designed to keep essential information in one convenient spot, whether you are tracking health vitals, organizing personal documents, or keeping track of your passwords. By following the steps below, you will ensure that you and anyone who may need to help you in an emergency can find critical information quickly and efficiently.

1. **Keep your information current**.
   Regularly update each section with current information or changes in your life. For example, if your prescription changes or you obtain new insurance, correct it immediately.

2. **Record Daily Medical Vitals**
   If you are monitoring health metrics, fill in the date and time for each entry. Consistently logging these vitals creates a clear health snapshot that could guide doctors in diagnosing conditions, adjusting treatments, and recommending lifestyle changes. Each page holds one week of vitals. If you need a logbook for more than medical information, such as passwords and logins, you can purchase an All-in-One Logbook from us on the platform of your choice.

3. **Track Medications and Allergies**
   Use a dedicated section to list your medication names, dosages, and schedules. Note any missed doses or side effects. You can also note any allergies and any medical alerts that you may have. Clearly mark any life-threatening allergies

with bold or highlight the text. Include details about the allergic reaction and the usual treatment.

4. **Keep a Medical Journal and Schedule Regular Doctor Visits**
Be sure to track daily symptoms, note how you are feeling, or record any new health questions. Bring this section to each doctor appointment to reference changes in vital signs or medications. Regular checkups help catch potential health issues early and keep treatments on the right track.

5. **Organize Important Documents and Contacts**
Gather details such as:
<u>Emergency Contacts</u>: Family, friends, neighbors, or any primary caregiver.
<u>Legal and Insurance Documents</u>: Wills, power of attorney, insurance policies, and important account information.

6. **Make Security a Priority**
Because this logbook contains sensitive information, consider storing it safely in a locked drawer or safe. For passwords and critical financial information, record only reminders or partial data.

7. **Review and Refine**
Once a month, or whenever information changes, review each section to see if anything needs updating. A quick monthly check ensures that your logbook remains a reliable, go to resource.

Storing these details in one location can be paramount when quick decisions or information is needed, especially during emergencies or natural disasters. By following these steps, you will make the most of your Medical Logbook, covering everything from daily vitals and medication updates to managing important documents and appointments, essentially giving you the tools to stay organized and proactive.

General Information

Name _____

Date of Birth _____

Gender _____

Home Phone _____

Cell Phone _____

Address _____

Email _____

Blood Type _____

Organ Donor _____

Preferred Hospital _____

Living Will _____

DNR on file _____

Communication Barrier _____

Other: _____

_____

_____

_____

Emergency Contacts

Name	Relationship	Phone Number	Email

Medical Alerts for Allergies

Allergen Name	Reaction	Severity	Treatment

Medical Conditions Alerts

Chronic Illness	Relevant Diagnoses	Surgical Implant/Device

<u>Doctor Information</u>   Primary Care Provider _____

Doctor Name	Specialty	Phone Number	Office Location

Medication Information   Pharmacy _____

Name	Amount	How Often	Purpose	Duration

Medical Visits

Date	Time	Doctor	Purpose/Topics to Discuss	Follow up?

Personal Vitals Importance

By consistently recording your vitals, complete with date and time, you'll create a clear snapshot of your day-to-day health, providing physicians with another resource to diagnose conditions, evaluate treatments, and recommend lifestyle modifications that can optimize your well-being.

Date & Time
Why It Matters: Recording the exact date and time ensures that any changes in your health can be linked to specific events or routines, such as recent meals, medication schedules, or sleep patterns. This context allows your doctor to spot trends, correlate symptoms with daily activities, and see if timing (morning vs. evening) affects your vital signs.

Blood Pressure
Why It Matters: Blood pressure readings give key insights into cardiovascular health. Hypertension (high blood pressure) can lead to serious complications if left uncontrolled, while low blood pressure may signal other issues. By logging blood pressure regularly, doctors can determine if treatments or lifestyle changes are effective, detect fluctuations that might require medication adjustments, and prevent long-term damage to the heart and blood vessels.

Heart Rate (Pulse)
Why It Matters: Your heart rate indicates how efficiently your heart is working and can reveal signs of stress or cardiac problems. An irregular or consistently high resting heart rate might suggest an underlying condition that needs attention. Tracking your pulse also

helps assess how well certain medications, like beta-blockers, are regulating your heart's workload.

Respiration Rate

Why It Matters: The number of breaths you take per minute can reflect respiratory function and overall wellness. An elevated rate might point to infection, anxiety, or lung/cardiac issues, while a low rate could be related to certain medications or underlying health conditions. Consistent recordings help doctors see if breathing patterns change over time or in response to medications.

Oxygen Level (SpO$_2$)

Why It Matters: Oxygen saturation levels show how effectively your lungs are transferring oxygen into your bloodstream. Low readings can alert you and your doctor to respiratory problems such as chronic obstructive pulmonary disease (COPD), asthma, or even cardiac issues. Tracking trends helps ensure that any drop in oxygen levels is promptly addressed and managed.

Blood Sugar (If needed)

Why It Matters: For individuals with diabetes or pre-diabetes, monitoring blood glucose levels is essential to prevent spikes (hyperglycemia) or dangerous drops (hypoglycemia). Charting these measurements over time reveals which meals, activities, or medications influence blood sugar most, allowing you and your healthcare team to adjust diet, exercise, or treatment plans for better control.

Weight

Why It Matters: Regular weigh-ins help detect trends in overall health, unexpected gain might suggest fluid retention (as in heart or kidney issues), while unwanted weight loss can indicate nutritional gaps or metabolic problems. By keeping a consistent record, you and your doctor can catch subtle changes early and respond with targeted advice or interventions.

Temperature

Why It Matters: Body temperature offers clues about infections, inflammation, or other medical conditions. A consistent low-grade fever or sudden spikes could point to emerging health concerns. Keeping track of temperature helps doctors see patterns, for instance, whether fevers occur at a certain time of day or coincide with other symptoms, and tailor diagnostic tests or treatments accordingly.

When you need more sheets, you can easily purchase another Medical Logbook from us on the platform of your choice.

Daily Vitals Log: *104 weeks = two full years*

Date	Time	Blood Pressure	Heart Rate	Resp Rate	Oxygen Level	Blood Sugar (Pre/Post/Fasting)	Weight	Temp
	__AM __PM	/				__Pre__Post__Fasting		

Symptoms/Notes:

Date	Time	Blood Pressure	Heart Rate	Resp Rate	Oxygen Level	Blood Sugar (Pre/Post/Fasting)	Weight	Temp
	__AM __PM	/				__Pre__Post__Fasting		

Symptoms/Notes:

Date	Time	Blood Pressure	Heart Rate	Resp Rate	Oxygen Level	Blood Sugar (Pre/Post/Fasting)	Weight	Temp
	__AM __PM	/				__Pre__Post__Fasting		

Symptoms/Notes:

Date	Time	Blood Pressure	Heart Rate	Resp Rate	Oxygen Level	Blood Sugar (Pre/Post/Fasting)	Weight	Temp
	__AM __PM	/				__Pre__Post__Fasting		

Symptoms/Notes:

Date	Time	Blood Pressure	Heart Rate	Resp Rate	Oxygen Level	Blood Sugar (Pre/Post/Fasting)	Weight	Temp
	__AM __PM	/				__Pre__Post__Fasting		

Symptoms/Notes:

Date	Time	Blood Pressure	Heart Rate	Resp Rate	Oxygen Level	Blood Sugar (Pre/Post/Fasting)	Weight	Temp
	__AM __PM	/				__Pre__Post__Fasting		

Symptoms/Notes:

Date	Time	Blood Pressure	Heart Rate	Resp Rate	Oxygen Level	Blood Sugar (Pre/Post/Fasting)	Weight	Temp
	__AM __PM	/				__Pre__Post__Fasting		

Symptoms/Notes:

Date	Time	Blood Pressure	Heart Rate	Resp Rate	Oxygen Level	Blood Sugar (Pre/Post/Fasting)	Weight	Temp
	__AM __PM	/				__Pre__Post__Fasting		

Symptoms/Notes:

Date	Time	Blood Pressure	Heart Rate	Resp Rate	Oxygen Level	Blood Sugar (Pre/Post/Fasting)	Weight	Temp
	__AM __PM	/				__Pre__Post__Fasting		

Symptoms/Notes:

Date	Time	Blood Pressure	Heart Rate	Resp Rate	Oxygen Level	Blood Sugar (Pre/Post/Fasting)	Weight	Temp
	__AM __PM	/				__Pre__Post__Fasting		

Symptoms/Notes:

Date	Time	Blood Pressure	Heart Rate	Resp Rate	Oxygen Level	Blood Sugar (Pre/Post/Fasting)	Weight	Temp
	__AM __PM	/				__Pre__Post__Fasting		

Symptoms/Notes:

Date	Time	Blood Pressure	Heart Rate	Resp Rate	Oxygen Level	Blood Sugar (Pre/Post/Fasting)	Weight	Temp
	__AM __PM	/				__Pre__Post__Fasting		

Symptoms/Notes:

Date	Time	Blood Pressure	Heart Rate	Resp Rate	Oxygen Level	Blood Sugar (Pre/Post/Fasting)	Weight	Temp
	__AM __PM	/				__Pre__Post__Fasting		

Symptoms/Notes:

Date	Time	Blood Pressure	Heart Rate	Resp Rate	Oxygen Level	Blood Sugar (Pre/Post/Fasting)	Weight	Temp
	__AM __PM	/				__Pre__Post__Fasting		

Symptoms/Notes:

Date	Time	Blood Pressure	Heart Rate	Resp Rate	Oxygen Level	Blood Sugar (Pre/Post/Fasting)	Weight	Temp
	__AM __PM	/				__Pre__Post__Fasting		

Symptoms/Notes:

Date	Time	Blood Pressure	Heart Rate	Resp Rate	Oxygen Level	Blood Sugar (Pre/Post/Fasting)	Weight	Temp
	__AM __PM	/				__Pre__Post__Fasting		

Symptoms/Notes:

Date	Time	Blood Pressure	Heart Rate	Resp Rate	Oxygen Level	Blood Sugar (Pre/Post/Fasting)	Weight	Temp
	__AM __PM	/				__Pre__Post__Fasting		

Symptoms/Notes:

Date	Time	Blood Pressure	Heart Rate	Resp Rate	Oxygen Level	Blood Sugar (Pre/Post/Fasting)	Weight	Temp
	__AM __PM	/				__Pre__Post__Fasting		

Symptoms/Notes:

Date	Time	Blood Pressure	Heart Rate	Resp Rate	Oxygen Level	Blood Sugar (Pre/Post/Fasting)	Weight	Temp
	__AM __PM	/				__Pre__Post__Fasting		

Symptoms/Notes:

Date	Time	Blood Pressure	Heart Rate	Resp Rate	Oxygen Level	Blood Sugar (Pre/Post/Fasting)	Weight	Temp
	__AM __PM	/				__Pre__Post__Fasting		

Symptoms/Notes:

Date	Time	Blood Pressure	Heart Rate	Resp Rate	Oxygen Level	Blood Sugar (Pre/Post/Fasting)	Weight	Temp
	__AM __PM	/				__Pre__Post__Fasting		

Symptoms/Notes:

Date	Time	Blood Pressure	Heart Rate	Resp Rate	Oxygen Level	Blood Sugar (Pre/Post/Fasting)	Weight	Temp
	__AM __PM	/				__Pre__Post__Fasting		

Symptoms/Notes:

Date	Time	Blood Pressure	Heart Rate	Resp Rate	Oxygen Level	Blood Sugar (Pre/Post/Fasting)	Weight	Temp
	__AM __PM	/				__Pre__Post__Fasting		

Symptoms/Notes:

Date	Time	Blood Pressure	Heart Rate	Resp Rate	Oxygen Level	Blood Sugar (Pre/Post/Fasting)	Weight	Temp
	__AM __PM	/				__Pre__Post__Fasting		

Symptoms/Notes:

Date	Time	Blood Pressure	Heart Rate	Resp Rate	Oxygen Level	Blood Sugar (Pre/Post/Fasting)	Weight	Temp
	__AM __PM	/				__Pre__Post__Fasting		

Symptoms/Notes:

Date	Time	Blood Pressure	Heart Rate	Resp Rate	Oxygen Level	Blood Sugar (Pre/Post/Fasting)	Weight	Temp
	__AM __PM	/				__Pre__Post__Fasting		

Symptoms/Notes:

Date	Time	Blood Pressure	Heart Rate	Resp Rate	Oxygen Level	Blood Sugar (Pre/Post/Fasting)	Weight	Temp
	__AM __PM	/				__Pre__Post__Fasting		

Symptoms/Notes:

Date	Time	Blood Pressure	Heart Rate	Resp Rate	Oxygen Level	Blood Sugar (Pre/Post/Fasting)	Weight	Temp
	__AM __PM	/				__Pre__Post__Fasting		

Symptoms/Notes:

Date	Time	Blood Pressure	Heart Rate	Resp Rate	Oxygen Level	Blood Sugar (Pre/Post/Fasting)	Weight	Temp
	__AM __PM	/				__Pre__Post__Fasting		

Symptoms/Notes:

Date	Time	Blood Pressure	Heart Rate	Resp Rate	Oxygen Level	Blood Sugar (Pre/Post/Fasting)	Weight	Temp
	__AM __PM	/				__Pre__Post__Fasting		

Symptoms/Notes:

Date	Time	Blood Pressure	Heart Rate	Resp Rate	Oxygen Level	Blood Sugar (Pre/Post/Fasting)	Weight	Temp
	__AM __PM	/				__Pre__Post__Fasting		

Symptoms/Notes:

Date	Time	Blood Pressure	Heart Rate	Resp Rate	Oxygen Level	Blood Sugar (Pre/Post/Fasting)	Weight	Temp
	__AM __PM	/				__Pre__Post__Fasting		

Symptoms/Notes:

Date	Time	Blood Pressure	Heart Rate	Resp Rate	Oxygen Level	Blood Sugar (Pre/Post/Fasting)	Weight	Temp
	__AM __PM	/				__Pre__Post__Fasting		

Symptoms/Notes:

Date	Time	Blood Pressure	Heart Rate	Resp Rate	Oxygen Level	Blood Sugar (Pre/Post/Fasting)	Weight	Temp
	__AM __PM	/				__Pre__Post__Fasting		

Symptoms/Notes:

Date	Time	Blood Pressure	Heart Rate	Resp Rate	Oxygen Level	Blood Sugar (Pre/Post/Fasting)	Weight	Temp
	__AM __PM	/				__Pre__Post__Fasting		

Symptoms/Notes:

Date	Time	Blood Pressure	Heart Rate	Resp Rate	Oxygen Level	Blood Sugar (Pre/Post/Fasting)	Weight	Temp
	__AM __PM	/				__Pre__Post__Fasting		

Symptoms/Notes:

Date	Time	Blood Pressure	Heart Rate	Resp Rate	Oxygen Level	Blood Sugar (Pre/Post/Fasting)	Weight	Temp
	__AM __PM	/				__Pre__Post__Fasting		

Symptoms/Notes:

Date	Time	Blood Pressure	Heart Rate	Resp Rate	Oxygen Level	Blood Sugar (Pre/Post/Fasting)	Weight	Temp
	__AM __PM	/				__Pre__Post__Fasting		

Symptoms/Notes:

Date	Time	Blood Pressure	Heart Rate	Resp Rate	Oxygen Level	Blood Sugar (Pre/Post/Fasting)	Weight	Temp
	__AM __PM	/				__Pre__Post__Fasting		

Symptoms/Notes:

Date	Time	Blood Pressure	Heart Rate	Resp Rate	Oxygen Level	Blood Sugar (Pre/Post/Fasting)	Weight	Temp
	__AM __PM	/				__Pre__Post__Fasting		

Symptoms/Notes:

Date	Time	Blood Pressure	Heart Rate	Resp Rate	Oxygen Level	Blood Sugar (Pre/Post/Fasting)	Weight	Temp
	__AM __PM	/				__Pre__Post__Fasting		

Symptoms/Notes:

Date	Time	Blood Pressure	Heart Rate	Resp Rate	Oxygen Level	Blood Sugar (Pre/Post/Fasting)	Weight	Temp
	__AM __PM	/				__Pre__Post__Fasting		

Symptoms/Notes:

Date	Time	Blood Pressure	Heart Rate	Resp Rate	Oxygen Level	Blood Sugar (Pre/Post/Fasting)	Weight	Temp
	__AM __PM	/				__Pre__Post__Fasting		

Symptoms/Notes:

Date	Time	Blood Pressure	Heart Rate	Resp Rate	Oxygen Level	Blood Sugar (Pre/Post/Fasting)	Weight	Temp
	__AM __PM	/				__Pre__Post__Fasting		

Symptoms/Notes:

Date	Time	Blood Pressure	Heart Rate	Resp Rate	Oxygen Level	Blood Sugar (Pre/Post/Fasting)	Weight	Temp
	__AM __PM	/				__Pre__Post__Fasting		

Symptoms/Notes:

Date	Time	Blood Pressure	Heart Rate	Resp Rate	Oxygen Level	Blood Sugar (Pre/Post/Fasting)	Weight	Temp
	__AM __PM	/				__Pre__Post__Fasting		

Symptoms/Notes:

Date	Time	Blood Pressure	Heart Rate	Resp Rate	Oxygen Level	Blood Sugar (Pre/Post/Fasting)	Weight	Temp
	__AM __PM	/				__Pre__Post__Fasting		

Symptoms/Notes:

Date	Time	Blood Pressure	Heart Rate	Resp Rate	Oxygen Level	Blood Sugar (Pre/Post/Fasting)	Weight	Temp
	__AM __PM	/				__Pre__Post__Fasting		

Symptoms/Notes:

Date	Time	Blood Pressure	Heart Rate	Resp Rate	Oxygen Level	Blood Sugar (Pre/Post/Fasting)	Weight	Temp
	__AM __PM	/				__Pre__Post__Fasting		

Symptoms/Notes:

Date	Time	Blood Pressure	Heart Rate	Resp Rate	Oxygen Level	Blood Sugar (Pre/Post/Fasting)	Weight	Temp
	__AM __PM	/				__Pre__Post__Fasting		

Symptoms/Notes:

Date	Time	Blood Pressure	Heart Rate	Resp Rate	Oxygen Level	Blood Sugar (Pre/Post/Fasting)	Weight	Temp
	__AM __PM	/				__Pre__Post__Fasting		

Symptoms/Notes:

Date	Time	Blood Pressure	Heart Rate	Resp Rate	Oxygen Level	Blood Sugar (Pre/Post/Fasting)	Weight	Temp
	__AM __PM	/				__Pre__Post__Fasting		

Symptoms/Notes:

Date	Time	Blood Pressure	Heart Rate	Resp Rate	Oxygen Level	Blood Sugar (Pre/Post/Fasting)	Weight	Temp
	__AM __PM	/				__Pre__Post__Fasting		

Symptoms/Notes:

Date	Time	Blood Pressure	Heart Rate	Resp Rate	Oxygen Level	Blood Sugar (Pre/Post/Fasting)	Weight	Temp
	__AM __PM	/				__Pre__Post__Fasting		

Symptoms/Notes:

Date	Time	Blood Pressure	Heart Rate	Resp Rate	Oxygen Level	Blood Sugar (Pre/Post/Fasting)	Weight	Temp
	__AM __PM	/				__Pre__Post__Fasting		

Symptoms/Notes:

Date	Time	Blood Pressure	Heart Rate	Resp Rate	Oxygen Level	Blood Sugar (Pre/Post/Fasting)	Weight	Temp
	__AM __PM	/				__Pre__Post__Fasting		

Symptoms/Notes:

Date	Time	Blood Pressure	Heart Rate	Resp Rate	Oxygen Level	Blood Sugar (Pre/Post/Fasting)	Weight	Temp
	__AM __PM	/				__Pre__Post__Fasting		

Symptoms/Notes:

Date	Time	Blood Pressure	Heart Rate	Resp Rate	Oxygen Level	Blood Sugar (Pre/Post/Fasting)	Weight	Temp
	__AM __PM	/				__Pre__Post__Fasting		

Symptoms/Notes:

Date	Time	Blood Pressure	Heart Rate	Resp Rate	Oxygen Level	Blood Sugar (Pre/Post/Fasting)	Weight	Temp
	__AM __PM	/				__Pre__Post__Fasting		

Symptoms/Notes:

Date	Time	Blood Pressure	Heart Rate	Resp Rate	Oxygen Level	Blood Sugar (Pre/Post/Fasting)	Weight	Temp
	__AM __PM	/				__Pre__Post__Fasting		

Symptoms/Notes:

Date	Time	Blood Pressure	Heart Rate	Resp Rate	Oxygen Level	Blood Sugar (Pre/Post/Fasting)	Weight	Temp
	__AM __PM	/				__Pre__Post__Fasting		

Symptoms/Notes:

Date	Time	Blood Pressure	Heart Rate	Resp Rate	Oxygen Level	Blood Sugar (Pre/Post/Fasting)	Weight	Temp
	__AM __PM	/				__Pre__Post__Fasting		

Symptoms/Notes:

Date	Time	Blood Pressure	Heart Rate	Resp Rate	Oxygen Level	Blood Sugar (Pre/Post/Fasting)	Weight	Temp
	__AM __PM	/				__Pre__Post__Fasting		

Symptoms/Notes:

Date	Time	Blood Pressure	Heart Rate	Resp Rate	Oxygen Level	Blood Sugar (Pre/Post/Fasting)	Weight	Temp
	__AM __PM	/				__Pre__Post__Fasting		

Symptoms/Notes:

Date	Time	Blood Pressure	Heart Rate	Resp Rate	Oxygen Level	Blood Sugar (Pre/Post/Fasting)	Weight	Temp
	__AM __PM	/				__Pre__Post__Fasting		

Symptoms/Notes:

Date	Time	Blood Pressure	Heart Rate	Resp Rate	Oxygen Level	Blood Sugar (Pre/Post/Fasting)	Weight	Temp
	__AM __PM	/				__Pre__Post__Fasting		

Symptoms/Notes:

Date	Time	Blood Pressure	Heart Rate	Resp Rate	Oxygen Level	Blood Sugar (Pre/Post/Fasting)	Weight	Temp
	__AM __PM	/				__Pre__Post__Fasting		

Symptoms/Notes:

Date	Time	Blood Pressure	Heart Rate	Resp Rate	Oxygen Level	Blood Sugar (Pre/Post/Fasting)	Weight	Temp
	__AM __PM	/				__Pre__Post__Fasting		

Symptoms/Notes:

Date	Time	Blood Pressure	Heart Rate	Resp Rate	Oxygen Level	Blood Sugar (Pre/Post/Fasting)	Weight	Temp
	__AM __PM	/				__Pre__Post__Fasting		

Symptoms/Notes:

Date	Time	Blood Pressure	Heart Rate	Resp Rate	Oxygen Level	Blood Sugar (Pre/Post/Fasting)	Weight	Temp
	__AM __PM	/				__Pre__Post__Fasting		

Symptoms/Notes:

Date	Time	Blood Pressure	Heart Rate	Resp Rate	Oxygen Level	Blood Sugar (Pre/Post/Fasting)	Weight	Temp
	__AM __PM	/				__Pre__Post__Fasting		

Symptoms/Notes:

Date	Time	Blood Pressure	Heart Rate	Resp Rate	Oxygen Level	Blood Sugar (Pre/Post/Fasting)	Weight	Temp
	__AM __PM	/				__Pre__Post__Fasting		

Symptoms/Notes:

Date	Time	Blood Pressure	Heart Rate	Resp Rate	Oxygen Level	Blood Sugar (Pre/Post/Fasting)	Weight	Temp
	__AM __PM	/				__Pre__Post__Fasting		

Symptoms/Notes:

Date	Time	Blood Pressure	Heart Rate	Resp Rate	Oxygen Level	Blood Sugar (Pre/Post/Fasting)	Weight	Temp
	__AM __PM	/				__Pre__Post__Fasting		

Symptoms/Notes:

Date	Time	Blood Pressure	Heart Rate	Resp Rate	Oxygen Level	Blood Sugar (Pre/Post/Fasting)	Weight	Temp
	__AM __PM	/				__Pre__Post__Fasting		

Symptoms/Notes:

Date	Time	Blood Pressure	Heart Rate	Resp Rate	Oxygen Level	Blood Sugar (Pre/Post/Fasting)	Weight	Temp
	__AM __PM	/				__Pre__Post__Fasting		

Symptoms/Notes:

Date	Time	Blood Pressure	Heart Rate	Resp Rate	Oxygen Level	Blood Sugar (Pre/Post/Fasting)	Weight	Temp
	__AM __PM	/				__Pre__Post__Fasting		

Symptoms/Notes:

Date	Time	Blood Pressure	Heart Rate	Resp Rate	Oxygen Level	Blood Sugar (Pre/Post/Fasting)	Weight	Temp
	__AM __PM	/				__Pre__Post__Fasting		

Symptoms/Notes:

Date	Time	Blood Pressure	Heart Rate	Resp Rate	Oxygen Level	Blood Sugar (Pre/Post/Fasting)	Weight	Temp
	__AM __PM	/				__Pre__Post__Fasting		

Symptoms/Notes:

Date	Time	Blood Pressure	Heart Rate	Resp Rate	Oxygen Level	Blood Sugar (Pre/Post/Fasting)	Weight	Temp
	__AM __PM	/				__Pre__Post__Fasting		

Symptoms/Notes:

Date	Time	Blood Pressure	Heart Rate	Resp Rate	Oxygen Level	Blood Sugar (Pre/Post/Fasting)	Weight	Temp
	__AM __PM	/				__Pre__Post__Fasting		

Symptoms/Notes:

Date	Time	Blood Pressure	Heart Rate	Resp Rate	Oxygen Level	Blood Sugar (Pre/Post/Fasting)	Weight	Temp
	__AM __PM	/				__Pre__Post__Fasting		

Symptoms/Notes:

Date	Time	Blood Pressure	Heart Rate	Resp Rate	Oxygen Level	Blood Sugar (Pre/Post/Fasting)	Weight	Temp
	__AM __PM	/				__Pre__Post__Fasting		

Symptoms/Notes:

Date	Time	Blood Pressure	Heart Rate	Resp Rate	Oxygen Level	Blood Sugar (Pre/Post/Fasting)	Weight	Temp
	__AM __PM	/				__Pre__Post__Fasting		

Symptoms/Notes:

Date	Time	Blood Pressure	Heart Rate	Resp Rate	Oxygen Level	Blood Sugar (Pre/Post/Fasting)	Weight	Temp
	__AM __PM	/				__Pre__Post__Fasting		

Symptoms/Notes:

Date	Time	Blood Pressure	Heart Rate	Resp Rate	Oxygen Level	Blood Sugar (Pre/Post/Fasting)	Weight	Temp
	__AM __PM	/				__Pre__Post__Fasting		

Symptoms/Notes:

Date	Time	Blood Pressure	Heart Rate	Resp Rate	Oxygen Level	Blood Sugar (Pre/Post/Fasting)	Weight	Temp
	__AM __PM	/				__Pre__Post__Fasting		

Symptoms/Notes:

Date	Time	Blood Pressure	Heart Rate	Resp Rate	Oxygen Level	Blood Sugar (Pre/Post/Fasting)	Weight	Temp
	__AM __PM	/				__Pre__Post__Fasting		

Symptoms/Notes:

Date	Time	Blood Pressure	Heart Rate	Resp Rate	Oxygen Level	Blood Sugar (Pre/Post/Fasting)	Weight	Temp
	__AM __PM	/				__Pre__Post__Fasting		

Symptoms/Notes:

Date	Time	Blood Pressure	Heart Rate	Resp Rate	Oxygen Level	Blood Sugar (Pre/Post/Fasting)	Weight	Temp
	__AM __PM	/				__Pre__Post__Fasting		

Symptoms/Notes:

Date	Time	Blood Pressure	Heart Rate	Resp Rate	Oxygen Level	Blood Sugar (Pre/Post/Fasting)	Weight	Temp
	__AM __PM	/				__Pre__Post__Fasting		

Symptoms/Notes:

Date	Time	Blood Pressure	Heart Rate	Resp Rate	Oxygen Level	Blood Sugar (Pre/Post/Fasting)	Weight	Temp
	__AM __PM	/				__Pre__Post__Fasting		

Symptoms/Notes:

Date	Time	Blood Pressure	Heart Rate	Resp Rate	Oxygen Level	Blood Sugar (Pre/Post/Fasting)	Weight	Temp
	__AM __PM	/				__Pre__Post__Fasting		

Symptoms/Notes:

Date	Time	Blood Pressure	Heart Rate	Resp Rate	Oxygen Level	Blood Sugar (Pre/Post/Fasting)	Weight	Temp
	__AM __PM	/				__Pre__Post__Fasting		

Symptoms/Notes:

Date	Time	Blood Pressure	Heart Rate	Resp Rate	Oxygen Level	Blood Sugar (Pre/Post/Fasting)	Weight	Temp
	__AM __PM	/				__Pre__Post__Fasting		

Symptoms/Notes:

Date	Time	Blood Pressure	Heart Rate	Resp Rate	Oxygen Level	Blood Sugar (Pre/Post/Fasting)	Weight	Temp
	__AM __PM	/				__Pre__Post__Fasting		

Symptoms/Notes:

Date	Time	Blood Pressure	Heart Rate	Resp Rate	Oxygen Level	Blood Sugar (Pre/Post/Fasting)	Weight	Temp
	__AM __PM	/				__Pre__Post__Fasting		

Symptoms/Notes:

Date	Time	Blood Pressure	Heart Rate	Resp Rate	Oxygen Level	Blood Sugar (Pre/Post/Fasting)	Weight	Temp
	__AM __PM	/				__Pre__Post__Fasting		

Symptoms/Notes:

Date	Time	Blood Pressure	Heart Rate	Resp Rate	Oxygen Level	Blood Sugar (Pre/Post/Fasting)	Weight	Temp
	__AM __PM	/				__Pre__Post__Fasting		

Symptoms/Notes:

Date	Time	Blood Pressure	Heart Rate	Resp Rate	Oxygen Level	Blood Sugar (Pre/Post/Fasting)	Weight	Temp
	__AM __PM	/				__Pre__Post__Fasting		

Symptoms/Notes:

Date	Time	Blood Pressure	Heart Rate	Resp Rate	Oxygen Level	Blood Sugar (Pre/Post/Fasting)	Weight	Temp
	__AM __PM	/				__Pre__Post__Fasting		

Symptoms/Notes:

Date	Time	Blood Pressure	Heart Rate	Resp Rate	Oxygen Level	Blood Sugar (Pre/Post/Fasting)	Weight	Temp
	__AM __PM	/				__Pre__Post__Fasting		

Symptoms/Notes:

Date	Time	Blood Pressure	Heart Rate	Resp Rate	Oxygen Level	Blood Sugar (Pre/Post/Fasting)	Weight	Temp
	__AM __PM	/				__Pre__Post__Fasting		

Symptoms/Notes:

Date	Time	Blood Pressure	Heart Rate	Resp Rate	Oxygen Level	Blood Sugar (Pre/Post/Fasting)	Weight	Temp
	__AM __PM	/				__Pre__Post__Fasting		

Symptoms/Notes:

Date	Time	Blood Pressure	Heart Rate	Resp Rate	Oxygen Level	Blood Sugar (Pre/Post/Fasting)	Weight	Temp
	__AM __PM	/				__Pre__Post__Fasting		

Symptoms/Notes:

Date	Time	Blood Pressure	Heart Rate	Resp Rate	Oxygen Level	Blood Sugar (Pre/Post/Fasting)	Weight	Temp
	__AM __PM	/				__Pre__Post__Fasting		

Symptoms/Notes:

Date	Time	Blood Pressure	Heart Rate	Resp Rate	Oxygen Level	Blood Sugar (Pre/Post/Fasting)	Weight	Temp
	__AM __PM	/				__Pre__Post__Fasting		

Symptoms/Notes:

Date	Time	Blood Pressure	Heart Rate	Resp Rate	Oxygen Level	Blood Sugar (Pre/Post/Fasting)	Weight	Temp
	__AM __PM	/				__Pre__Post__Fasting		

Symptoms/Notes:

Date	Time	Blood Pressure	Heart Rate	Resp Rate	Oxygen Level	Blood Sugar (Pre/Post/Fasting)	Weight	Temp
	__AM __PM	/				__Pre__Post__Fasting		

Symptoms/Notes:

Date	Time	Blood Pressure	Heart Rate	Resp Rate	Oxygen Level	Blood Sugar (Pre/Post/Fasting)	Weight	Temp
	__AM __PM	/				__Pre__Post__Fasting		

Symptoms/Notes:

Date	Time	Blood Pressure	Heart Rate	Resp Rate	Oxygen Level	Blood Sugar (Pre/Post/Fasting)	Weight	Temp
	__AM __PM	/				__Pre__Post__Fasting		

Symptoms/Notes:

Date	Time	Blood Pressure	Heart Rate	Resp Rate	Oxygen Level	Blood Sugar (Pre/Post/Fasting)	Weight	Temp
	__AM __PM	/				__Pre__Post__Fasting		

Symptoms/Notes:

Date	Time	Blood Pressure	Heart Rate	Resp Rate	Oxygen Level	Blood Sugar (Pre/Post/Fasting)	Weight	Temp
	__AM __PM	/				__Pre__Post__Fasting		

Symptoms/Notes:

Date	Time	Blood Pressure	Heart Rate	Resp Rate	Oxygen Level	Blood Sugar (Pre/Post/Fasting)	Weight	Temp
	__AM __PM	/				__Pre__Post__Fasting		

Symptoms/Notes:

Date	Time	Blood Pressure	Heart Rate	Resp Rate	Oxygen Level	Blood Sugar (Pre/Post/Fasting)	Weight	Temp
	__AM __PM	/				__Pre__Post__Fasting		

Symptoms/Notes:

Date	Time	Blood Pressure	Heart Rate	Resp Rate	Oxygen Level	Blood Sugar (Pre/Post/Fasting)	Weight	Temp
	__AM __PM	/				__Pre__Post__Fasting		

Symptoms/Notes:

Date	Time	Blood Pressure	Heart Rate	Resp Rate	Oxygen Level	Blood Sugar (Pre/Post/Fasting)	Weight	Temp
	__AM __PM	/				__Pre__Post__Fasting		

Symptoms/Notes:

Date	Time	Blood Pressure	Heart Rate	Resp Rate	Oxygen Level	Blood Sugar (Pre/Post/Fasting)	Weight	Temp
	__AM __PM	/				__Pre__Post__Fasting		

Symptoms/Notes:

Date	Time	Blood Pressure	Heart Rate	Resp Rate	Oxygen Level	Blood Sugar (Pre/Post/Fasting)	Weight	Temp
	__AM __PM	/				__Pre__Post__Fasting		

Symptoms/Notes:

Date	Time	Blood Pressure	Heart Rate	Resp Rate	Oxygen Level	Blood Sugar (Pre/Post/Fasting)	Weight	Temp
	__AM __PM	/				__Pre__Post__Fasting		

Symptoms/Notes:

Date	Time	Blood Pressure	Heart Rate	Resp Rate	Oxygen Level	Blood Sugar (Pre/Post/Fasting)	Weight	Temp
	__AM __PM	/				__Pre__Post__Fasting		

Symptoms/Notes:

Date	Time	Blood Pressure	Heart Rate	Resp Rate	Oxygen Level	Blood Sugar (Pre/Post/Fasting)	Weight	Temp
	__AM __PM	/				__Pre__Post__Fasting		

Symptoms/Notes:

Date	Time	Blood Pressure	Heart Rate	Resp Rate	Oxygen Level	Blood Sugar (Pre/Post/Fasting)	Weight	Temp
	__AM __PM	/				__Pre__Post__Fasting		

Symptoms/Notes:

Date	Time	Blood Pressure	Heart Rate	Resp Rate	Oxygen Level	Blood Sugar (Pre/Post/Fasting)	Weight	Temp
	__AM __PM	/				__Pre__Post__Fasting		

Symptoms/Notes:

Date	Time	Blood Pressure	Heart Rate	Resp Rate	Oxygen Level	Blood Sugar (Pre/Post/Fasting)	Weight	Temp
	__AM __PM	/				__Pre__Post__Fasting		

Symptoms/Notes:

Date	Time	Blood Pressure	Heart Rate	Resp Rate	Oxygen Level	Blood Sugar (Pre/Post/Fasting)	Weight	Temp
	__AM __PM	/				__Pre__Post__Fasting		

Symptoms/Notes:

Date	Time	Blood Pressure	Heart Rate	Resp Rate	Oxygen Level	Blood Sugar (Pre/Post/Fasting)	Weight	Temp
	__AM __PM	/				__Pre __Post __Fasting		

Symptoms/Notes:

Date	Time	Blood Pressure	Heart Rate	Resp Rate	Oxygen Level	Blood Sugar (Pre/Post/Fasting)	Weight	Temp
	__AM __PM	/				__Pre __Post __Fasting		

Symptoms/Notes:

Date	Time	Blood Pressure	Heart Rate	Resp Rate	Oxygen Level	Blood Sugar (Pre/Post/Fasting)	Weight	Temp
	__AM __PM	/				__Pre __Post __Fasting		

Symptoms/Notes:

Date	Time	Blood Pressure	Heart Rate	Resp Rate	Oxygen Level	Blood Sugar (Pre/Post/Fasting)	Weight	Temp
	__AM __PM	/				__Pre __Post __Fasting		

Symptoms/Notes:

Date	Time	Blood Pressure	Heart Rate	Resp Rate	Oxygen Level	Blood Sugar (Pre/Post/Fasting)	Weight	Temp
	__AM __PM	/				__Pre __Post __Fasting		

Symptoms/Notes:

Date	Time	Blood Pressure	Heart Rate	Resp Rate	Oxygen Level	Blood Sugar (Pre/Post/Fasting)	Weight	Temp
	__AM __PM	/				__Pre __Post __Fasting		

Symptoms/Notes:

Date	Time	Blood Pressure	Heart Rate	Resp Rate	Oxygen Level	Blood Sugar (Pre/Post/Fasting)	Weight	Temp
	__AM __PM	/				__Pre __Post __Fasting		

Symptoms/Notes:

Date	Time	Blood Pressure	Heart Rate	Resp Rate	Oxygen Level	Blood Sugar (Pre/Post/Fasting)	Weight	Temp
	__AM __PM	/				__Pre__Post__Fasting		

Symptoms/Notes:

Date	Time	Blood Pressure	Heart Rate	Resp Rate	Oxygen Level	Blood Sugar (Pre/Post/Fasting)	Weight	Temp
	__AM __PM	/				__Pre__Post__Fasting		

Symptoms/Notes:

Date	Time	Blood Pressure	Heart Rate	Resp Rate	Oxygen Level	Blood Sugar (Pre/Post/Fasting)	Weight	Temp
	__AM __PM	/				__Pre__Post__Fasting		

Symptoms/Notes:

Date	Time	Blood Pressure	Heart Rate	Resp Rate	Oxygen Level	Blood Sugar (Pre/Post/Fasting)	Weight	Temp
	__AM __PM	/				__Pre__Post__Fasting		

Symptoms/Notes:

Date	Time	Blood Pressure	Heart Rate	Resp Rate	Oxygen Level	Blood Sugar (Pre/Post/Fasting)	Weight	Temp
	__AM __PM	/				__Pre__Post__Fasting		

Symptoms/Notes:

Date	Time	Blood Pressure	Heart Rate	Resp Rate	Oxygen Level	Blood Sugar (Pre/Post/Fasting)	Weight	Temp
	__AM __PM	/				__Pre__Post__Fasting		

Symptoms/Notes:

Date	Time	Blood Pressure	Heart Rate	Resp Rate	Oxygen Level	Blood Sugar (Pre/Post/Fasting)	Weight	Temp
	__AM __PM	/				__Pre__Post__Fasting		

Symptoms/Notes:

Date	Time	Blood Pressure	Heart Rate	Resp Rate	Oxygen Level	Blood Sugar (Pre/Post/Fasting)	Weight	Temp
	__AM __PM	/				__Pre__Post__Fasting		

Symptoms/Notes:

Date	Time	Blood Pressure	Heart Rate	Resp Rate	Oxygen Level	Blood Sugar (Pre/Post/Fasting)	Weight	Temp
	__AM __PM	/				__Pre__Post__Fasting		

Symptoms/Notes:

Date	Time	Blood Pressure	Heart Rate	Resp Rate	Oxygen Level	Blood Sugar (Pre/Post/Fasting)	Weight	Temp
	__AM __PM	/				__Pre__Post__Fasting		

Symptoms/Notes:

Date	Time	Blood Pressure	Heart Rate	Resp Rate	Oxygen Level	Blood Sugar (Pre/Post/Fasting)	Weight	Temp
	__AM __PM	/				__Pre__Post__Fasting		

Symptoms/Notes:

Date	Time	Blood Pressure	Heart Rate	Resp Rate	Oxygen Level	Blood Sugar (Pre/Post/Fasting)	Weight	Temp
	__AM __PM	/				__Pre__Post__Fasting		

Symptoms/Notes:

Date	Time	Blood Pressure	Heart Rate	Resp Rate	Oxygen Level	Blood Sugar (Pre/Post/Fasting)	Weight	Temp
	__AM __PM	/				__Pre__Post__Fasting		

Symptoms/Notes:

Date	Time	Blood Pressure	Heart Rate	Resp Rate	Oxygen Level	Blood Sugar (Pre/Post/Fasting)	Weight	Temp
	__AM __PM	/				__Pre__Post__Fasting		

Symptoms/Notes:

Date	Time	Blood Pressure	Heart Rate	Resp Rate	Oxygen Level	Blood Sugar (Pre/Post/Fasting)	Weight	Temp
	__AM __PM	/				__Pre__Post__Fasting		

Symptoms/Notes:

Date	Time	Blood Pressure	Heart Rate	Resp Rate	Oxygen Level	Blood Sugar (Pre/Post/Fasting)	Weight	Temp
	__AM __PM	/				__Pre__Post__Fasting		

Symptoms/Notes:

Date	Time	Blood Pressure	Heart Rate	Resp Rate	Oxygen Level	Blood Sugar (Pre/Post/Fasting)	Weight	Temp
	__AM __PM	/				__Pre__Post__Fasting		

Symptoms/Notes:

Date	Time	Blood Pressure	Heart Rate	Resp Rate	Oxygen Level	Blood Sugar (Pre/Post/Fasting)	Weight	Temp
	__AM __PM	/				__Pre__Post__Fasting		

Symptoms/Notes:

Date	Time	Blood Pressure	Heart Rate	Resp Rate	Oxygen Level	Blood Sugar (Pre/Post/Fasting)	Weight	Temp
	__AM __PM	/				__Pre__Post__Fasting		

Symptoms/Notes:

Date	Time	Blood Pressure	Heart Rate	Resp Rate	Oxygen Level	Blood Sugar (Pre/Post/Fasting)	Weight	Temp
	__AM __PM	/				__Pre__Post__Fasting		

Symptoms/Notes:

Date	Time	Blood Pressure	Heart Rate	Resp Rate	Oxygen Level	Blood Sugar (Pre/Post/Fasting)	Weight	Temp
	__AM __PM	/				__Pre__Post__Fasting		

Symptoms/Notes:

Date	Time	Blood Pressure	Heart Rate	Resp Rate	Oxygen Level	Blood Sugar (Pre/Post/Fasting)	Weight	Temp
	__AM __PM	/				__Pre__Post__Fasting		

Symptoms/Notes:

Date	Time	Blood Pressure	Heart Rate	Resp Rate	Oxygen Level	Blood Sugar (Pre/Post/Fasting)	Weight	Temp
	__AM __PM	/				__Pre__Post__Fasting		

Symptoms/Notes:

Date	Time	Blood Pressure	Heart Rate	Resp Rate	Oxygen Level	Blood Sugar (Pre/Post/Fasting)	Weight	Temp
	__AM __PM	/				__Pre__Post__Fasting		

Symptoms/Notes:

Date	Time	Blood Pressure	Heart Rate	Resp Rate	Oxygen Level	Blood Sugar (Pre/Post/Fasting)	Weight	Temp
	__AM __PM	/				__Pre__Post__Fasting		

Symptoms/Notes:

Date	Time	Blood Pressure	Heart Rate	Resp Rate	Oxygen Level	Blood Sugar (Pre/Post/Fasting)	Weight	Temp
	__AM __PM	/				__Pre__Post__Fasting		

Symptoms/Notes:

Date	Time	Blood Pressure	Heart Rate	Resp Rate	Oxygen Level	Blood Sugar (Pre/Post/Fasting)	Weight	Temp
	__AM __PM	/				__Pre__Post__Fasting		

Symptoms/Notes:

Date	Time	Blood Pressure	Heart Rate	Resp Rate	Oxygen Level	Blood Sugar (Pre/Post/Fasting)	Weight	Temp
	__AM __PM	/				__Pre__Post__Fasting		

Symptoms/Notes:

Date	Time	Blood Pressure	Heart Rate	Resp Rate	Oxygen Level	Blood Sugar (Pre/Post/Fasting)	Weight	Temp
	__AM __PM	/				__Pre__Post__Fasting		

Symptoms/Notes:

Date	Time	Blood Pressure	Heart Rate	Resp Rate	Oxygen Level	Blood Sugar (Pre/Post/Fasting)	Weight	Temp
	__AM __PM	/				__Pre__Post__Fasting		

Symptoms/Notes:

Date	Time	Blood Pressure	Heart Rate	Resp Rate	Oxygen Level	Blood Sugar (Pre/Post/Fasting)	Weight	Temp
	__AM __PM	/				__Pre__Post__Fasting		

Symptoms/Notes:

Date	Time	Blood Pressure	Heart Rate	Resp Rate	Oxygen Level	Blood Sugar (Pre/Post/Fasting)	Weight	Temp
	__AM __PM	/				__Pre__Post__Fasting		

Symptoms/Notes:

Date	Time	Blood Pressure	Heart Rate	Resp Rate	Oxygen Level	Blood Sugar (Pre/Post/Fasting)	Weight	Temp
	__AM __PM	/				__Pre__Post__Fasting		

Symptoms/Notes:

Date	Time	Blood Pressure	Heart Rate	Resp Rate	Oxygen Level	Blood Sugar (Pre/Post/Fasting)	Weight	Temp
	__AM __PM	/				__Pre__Post__Fasting		

Symptoms/Notes:

Date	Time	Blood Pressure	Heart Rate	Resp Rate	Oxygen Level	Blood Sugar (Pre/Post/Fasting)	Weight	Temp
	__AM __PM	/				__Pre__Post__Fasting		

Symptoms/Notes:

Date	Time	Blood Pressure	Heart Rate	Resp Rate	Oxygen Level	Blood Sugar (Pre/Post/Fasting)	Weight	Temp
	__AM __PM	/				__Pre__Post__Fasting		

Symptoms/Notes:

Date	Time	Blood Pressure	Heart Rate	Resp Rate	Oxygen Level	Blood Sugar (Pre/Post/Fasting)	Weight	Temp
	__AM __PM	/				__Pre__Post__Fasting		

Symptoms/Notes:

Date	Time	Blood Pressure	Heart Rate	Resp Rate	Oxygen Level	Blood Sugar (Pre/Post/Fasting)	Weight	Temp
	__AM __PM	/				__Pre__Post__Fasting		

Symptoms/Notes:

Date	Time	Blood Pressure	Heart Rate	Resp Rate	Oxygen Level	Blood Sugar (Pre/Post/Fasting)	Weight	Temp
	__AM __PM	/				__Pre__Post__Fasting		

Symptoms/Notes:

Date	Time	Blood Pressure	Heart Rate	Resp Rate	Oxygen Level	Blood Sugar (Pre/Post/Fasting)	Weight	Temp
	__AM __PM	/				__Pre__Post__Fasting		

Symptoms/Notes:

Date	Time	Blood Pressure	Heart Rate	Resp Rate	Oxygen Level	Blood Sugar (Pre/Post/Fasting)	Weight	Temp
	__AM __PM	/				__Pre__Post__Fasting		

Symptoms/Notes:

Date	Time	Blood Pressure	Heart Rate	Resp Rate	Oxygen Level	Blood Sugar (Pre/Post/Fasting)	Weight	Temp
	__AM __PM	/				__Pre__Post__Fasting		

Symptoms/Notes:

Date	Time	Blood Pressure	Heart Rate	Resp Rate	Oxygen Level	Blood Sugar (Pre/Post/Fasting)	Weight	Temp
	__AM __PM	/				__Pre__Post__Fasting		

Symptoms/Notes:

Date	Time	Blood Pressure	Heart Rate	Resp Rate	Oxygen Level	Blood Sugar (Pre/Post/Fasting)	Weight	Temp
	__AM __PM	/				__Pre__Post__Fasting		

Symptoms/Notes:

Date	Time	Blood Pressure	Heart Rate	Resp Rate	Oxygen Level	Blood Sugar (Pre/Post/Fasting)	Weight	Temp
	__AM __PM	/				__Pre__Post__Fasting		

Symptoms/Notes:

Date	Time	Blood Pressure	Heart Rate	Resp Rate	Oxygen Level	Blood Sugar (Pre/Post/Fasting)	Weight	Temp
	__AM __PM	/				__Pre__Post__Fasting		

Symptoms/Notes:

Date	Time	Blood Pressure	Heart Rate	Resp Rate	Oxygen Level	Blood Sugar (Pre/Post/Fasting)	Weight	Temp
	__AM __PM	/				__Pre__Post__Fasting		

Symptoms/Notes:

Date	Time	Blood Pressure	Heart Rate	Resp Rate	Oxygen Level	Blood Sugar (Pre/Post/Fasting)	Weight	Temp
	__AM __PM	/				__Pre__Post__Fasting		

Symptoms/Notes:

Date	Time	Blood Pressure	Heart Rate	Resp Rate	Oxygen Level	Blood Sugar (Pre/Post/Fasting)	Weight	Temp
	__AM __PM	/				__Pre__Post__Fasting		

Symptoms/Notes:

Date	Time	Blood Pressure	Heart Rate	Resp Rate	Oxygen Level	Blood Sugar (Pre/Post/Fasting)	Weight	Temp
	__AM __PM	/				__Pre__Post__Fasting		

Symptoms/Notes:

Date	Time	Blood Pressure	Heart Rate	Resp Rate	Oxygen Level	Blood Sugar (Pre/Post/Fasting)	Weight	Temp
	__AM __PM	/				__Pre__Post__Fasting		

Symptoms/Notes:

Date	Time	Blood Pressure	Heart Rate	Resp Rate	Oxygen Level	Blood Sugar (Pre/Post/Fasting)	Weight	Temp
	__AM __PM	/				__Pre__Post__Fasting		

Symptoms/Notes:

Date	Time	Blood Pressure	Heart Rate	Resp Rate	Oxygen Level	Blood Sugar (Pre/Post/Fasting)	Weight	Temp
	__AM __PM	/				__Pre__Post__Fasting		

Symptoms/Notes:

Date	Time	Blood Pressure	Heart Rate	Resp Rate	Oxygen Level	Blood Sugar (Pre/Post/Fasting)	Weight	Temp
	__AM __PM	/				__Pre__Post__Fasting		

Symptoms/Notes:

Date	Time	Blood Pressure	Heart Rate	Resp Rate	Oxygen Level	Blood Sugar (Pre/Post/Fasting)	Weight	Temp
	__AM __PM	/				__Pre__Post__Fasting		

Symptoms/Notes:

Date	Time	Blood Pressure	Heart Rate	Resp Rate	Oxygen Level	Blood Sugar (Pre/Post/Fasting)	Weight	Temp
	__AM __PM	/				__Pre__Post__Fasting		

Symptoms/Notes:

Date	Time	Blood Pressure	Heart Rate	Resp Rate	Oxygen Level	Blood Sugar (Pre/Post/Fasting)	Weight	Temp
	__AM __PM	/				__Pre__Post__Fasting		

Symptoms/Notes:

Date	Time	Blood Pressure	Heart Rate	Resp Rate	Oxygen Level	Blood Sugar (Pre/Post/Fasting)	Weight	Temp
	__AM __PM	/				__Pre__Post__Fasting		

Symptoms/Notes:

Date	Time	Blood Pressure	Heart Rate	Resp Rate	Oxygen Level	Blood Sugar (Pre/Post/Fasting)	Weight	Temp
	__AM __PM	/				__Pre__Post__Fasting		

Symptoms/Notes:

Date	Time	Blood Pressure	Heart Rate	Resp Rate	Oxygen Level	Blood Sugar (Pre/Post/Fasting)	Weight	Temp
	__AM __PM	/				__Pre__Post__Fasting		

Symptoms/Notes:

Date	Time	Blood Pressure	Heart Rate	Resp Rate	Oxygen Level	Blood Sugar (Pre/Post/Fasting)	Weight	Temp
	__AM __PM	/				__Pre__Post__Fasting		

Symptoms/Notes:

Date	Time	Blood Pressure	Heart Rate	Resp Rate	Oxygen Level	Blood Sugar (Pre/Post/Fasting)	Weight	Temp
	__AM __PM	/				__Pre__Post__Fasting		

Symptoms/Notes:

Date	Time	Blood Pressure	Heart Rate	Resp Rate	Oxygen Level	Blood Sugar (Pre/Post/Fasting)	Weight	Temp
	__AM __PM	/				__Pre__Post__Fasting		

Symptoms/Notes:

Date	Time	Blood Pressure	Heart Rate	Resp Rate	Oxygen Level	Blood Sugar (Pre/Post/Fasting)	Weight	Temp
	__AM __PM	/				__Pre__Post__Fasting		

Symptoms/Notes:

Date	Time	Blood Pressure	Heart Rate	Resp Rate	Oxygen Level	Blood Sugar (Pre/Post/Fasting)	Weight	Temp
	__AM __PM	/				__Pre__Post__Fasting		

Symptoms/Notes:

Date	Time	Blood Pressure	Heart Rate	Resp Rate	Oxygen Level	Blood Sugar (Pre/Post/Fasting)	Weight	Temp
	__AM __PM	/				__Pre__Post__Fasting		

Symptoms/Notes:

Date	Time	Blood Pressure	Heart Rate	Resp Rate	Oxygen Level	Blood Sugar (Pre/Post/Fasting)	Weight	Temp
	__AM __PM	/				__Pre__Post__Fasting		

Symptoms/Notes:

Date	Time	Blood Pressure	Heart Rate	Resp Rate	Oxygen Level	Blood Sugar (Pre/Post/Fasting)	Weight	Temp
	__AM __PM	/				__Pre__Post__Fasting		

Symptoms/Notes:

Date	Time	Blood Pressure	Heart Rate	Resp Rate	Oxygen Level	Blood Sugar (Pre/Post/Fasting)	Weight	Temp
	__AM __PM	/				__Pre__Post__Fasting		

Symptoms/Notes:

Date	Time	Blood Pressure	Heart Rate	Resp Rate	Oxygen Level	Blood Sugar (Pre/Post/Fasting)	Weight	Temp
	__AM __PM	/				__Pre__Post__Fasting		

Symptoms/Notes:

Date	Time	Blood Pressure	Heart Rate	Resp Rate	Oxygen Level	Blood Sugar (Pre/Post/Fasting)	Weight	Temp
	__AM __PM	/				__Pre__Post__Fasting		

Symptoms/Notes:

Date	Time	Blood Pressure	Heart Rate	Resp Rate	Oxygen Level	Blood Sugar (Pre/Post/Fasting)	Weight	Temp
	__AM __PM	/				__Pre__Post__Fasting		

Symptoms/Notes:

Date	Time	Blood Pressure	Heart Rate	Resp Rate	Oxygen Level	Blood Sugar (Pre/Post/Fasting)	Weight	Temp
	__AM __PM	/				__Pre__Post__Fasting		

Symptoms/Notes:

Date	Time	Blood Pressure	Heart Rate	Resp Rate	Oxygen Level	Blood Sugar (Pre/Post/Fasting)	Weight	Temp
	__AM __PM	/				__Pre__Post__Fasting		

Symptoms/Notes:

Date	Time	Blood Pressure	Heart Rate	Resp Rate	Oxygen Level	Blood Sugar (Pre/Post/Fasting)	Weight	Temp
	__AM __PM	/				__Pre__Post__Fasting		

Symptoms/Notes:

Date	Time	Blood Pressure	Heart Rate	Resp Rate	Oxygen Level	Blood Sugar (Pre/Post/Fasting)	Weight	Temp
	__AM __PM	/				__Pre__Post__Fasting		

Symptoms/Notes:

Date	Time	Blood Pressure	Heart Rate	Resp Rate	Oxygen Level	Blood Sugar (Pre/Post/Fasting)	Weight	Temp
	__AM __PM	/				__Pre__Post__Fasting		

Symptoms/Notes:

Date	Time	Blood Pressure	Heart Rate	Resp Rate	Oxygen Level	Blood Sugar (Pre/Post/Fasting)	Weight	Temp
	__AM __PM	/				__Pre__Post__Fasting		

Symptoms/Notes:

Date	Time	Blood Pressure	Heart Rate	Resp Rate	Oxygen Level	Blood Sugar (Pre/Post/Fasting)	Weight	Temp
	__AM __PM	/				__Pre__Post__Fasting		

Symptoms/Notes:

Date	Time	Blood Pressure	Heart Rate	Resp Rate	Oxygen Level	Blood Sugar (Pre/Post/Fasting)	Weight	Temp
	__AM __PM	/				__Pre__Post__Fasting		

Symptoms/Notes:

Date	Time	Blood Pressure	Heart Rate	Resp Rate	Oxygen Level	Blood Sugar (Pre/Post/Fasting)	Weight	Temp
	__AM __PM	/				__Pre__Post__Fasting		

Symptoms/Notes:

Date	Time	Blood Pressure	Heart Rate	Resp Rate	Oxygen Level	Blood Sugar (Pre/Post/Fasting)	Weight	Temp
	__AM __PM	/				__Pre__Post__Fasting		

Symptoms/Notes:

Date	Time	Blood Pressure	Heart Rate	Resp Rate	Oxygen Level	Blood Sugar (Pre/Post/Fasting)	Weight	Temp
	__AM __PM	/				__Pre__Post__Fasting		

Symptoms/Notes:

Date	Time	Blood Pressure	Heart Rate	Resp Rate	Oxygen Level	Blood Sugar (Pre/Post/Fasting)	Weight	Temp
	__AM __PM	/				__Pre__Post__Fasting		

Symptoms/Notes:

Date	Time	Blood Pressure	Heart Rate	Resp Rate	Oxygen Level	Blood Sugar (Pre/Post/Fasting)	Weight	Temp
	__AM __PM	/				__Pre__Post__Fasting		

Symptoms/Notes:

Date	Time	Blood Pressure	Heart Rate	Resp Rate	Oxygen Level	Blood Sugar (Pre/Post/Fasting)	Weight	Temp
	__AM __PM	/				__Pre__Post__Fasting		

Symptoms/Notes:

Date	Time	Blood Pressure	Heart Rate	Resp Rate	Oxygen Level	Blood Sugar (Pre/Post/Fasting)	Weight	Temp
	__AM __PM	/				__Pre__Post__Fasting		

Symptoms/Notes:

Date	Time	Blood Pressure	Heart Rate	Resp Rate	Oxygen Level	Blood Sugar (Pre/Post/Fasting)	Weight	Temp
	__AM __PM	/				__Pre__Post__Fasting		

Symptoms/Notes:

Date	Time	Blood Pressure	Heart Rate	Resp Rate	Oxygen Level	Blood Sugar (Pre/Post/Fasting)	Weight	Temp
	__AM __PM	/				__Pre__Post__Fasting		

Symptoms/Notes:

Date	Time	Blood Pressure	Heart Rate	Resp Rate	Oxygen Level	Blood Sugar (Pre/Post/Fasting)	Weight	Temp
	__AM __PM	/				__Pre__Post__Fasting		

Symptoms/Notes:

Date	Time	Blood Pressure	Heart Rate	Resp Rate	Oxygen Level	Blood Sugar (Pre/Post/Fasting)	Weight	Temp
	__AM __PM	/				__Pre__Post__Fasting		

Symptoms/Notes:

Date	Time	Blood Pressure	Heart Rate	Resp Rate	Oxygen Level	Blood Sugar (Pre/Post/Fasting)	Weight	Temp
	__AM __PM	/				__Pre__Post__Fasting		

Symptoms/Notes:

Date	Time	Blood Pressure	Heart Rate	Resp Rate	Oxygen Level	Blood Sugar (Pre/Post/Fasting)	Weight	Temp
	__AM __PM	/				__Pre__Post__Fasting		

Symptoms/Notes:

Date	Time	Blood Pressure	Heart Rate	Resp Rate	Oxygen Level	Blood Sugar (Pre/Post/Fasting)	Weight	Temp
	__AM __PM	/				__Pre__Post__Fasting		

Symptoms/Notes:

Date	Time	Blood Pressure	Heart Rate	Resp Rate	Oxygen Level	Blood Sugar (Pre/Post/Fasting)	Weight	Temp
	__AM __PM	/				__Pre__Post__Fasting		

Symptoms/Notes:

Date	Time	Blood Pressure	Heart Rate	Resp Rate	Oxygen Level	Blood Sugar (Pre/Post/Fasting)	Weight	Temp
	__AM __PM	/				__Pre__Post__Fasting		

Symptoms/Notes:

Date	Time	Blood Pressure	Heart Rate	Resp Rate	Oxygen Level	Blood Sugar (Pre/Post/Fasting)	Weight	Temp
	__AM __PM	/				__Pre__Post__Fasting		

Symptoms/Notes:

Date	Time	Blood Pressure	Heart Rate	Resp Rate	Oxygen Level	Blood Sugar (Pre/Post/Fasting)	Weight	Temp
	__AM __PM	/				__Pre__Post__Fasting		

Symptoms/Notes:

Date	Time	Blood Pressure	Heart Rate	Resp Rate	Oxygen Level	Blood Sugar (Pre/Post/Fasting)	Weight	Temp
	__AM __PM	/				__Pre__Post__Fasting		

Symptoms/Notes:

Date	Time	Blood Pressure	Heart Rate	Resp Rate	Oxygen Level	Blood Sugar (Pre/Post/Fasting)	Weight	Temp
	__AM __PM	/				__Pre__Post__Fasting		

Symptoms/Notes:

Date	Time	Blood Pressure	Heart Rate	Resp Rate	Oxygen Level	Blood Sugar (Pre/Post/Fasting)	Weight	Temp
	__AM __PM	/				__Pre__Post__Fasting		

Symptoms/Notes:

Date	Time	Blood Pressure	Heart Rate	Resp Rate	Oxygen Level	Blood Sugar (Pre/Post/Fasting)	Weight	Temp
	__AM __PM	/				__Pre__Post__Fasting		

Symptoms/Notes:

Date	Time	Blood Pressure	Heart Rate	Resp Rate	Oxygen Level	Blood Sugar (Pre/Post/Fasting)	Weight	Temp
	__AM __PM	/				__Pre__Post__Fasting		

Symptoms/Notes:

Date	Time	Blood Pressure	Heart Rate	Resp Rate	Oxygen Level	Blood Sugar (Pre/Post/Fasting)	Weight	Temp
	__AM __PM	/				__Pre__Post__Fasting		

Symptoms/Notes:

Date	Time	Blood Pressure	Heart Rate	Resp Rate	Oxygen Level	Blood Sugar (Pre/Post/Fasting)	Weight	Temp
	__AM __PM	/				__Pre__Post__Fasting		

Symptoms/Notes:

Date	Time	Blood Pressure	Heart Rate	Resp Rate	Oxygen Level	Blood Sugar (Pre/Post/Fasting)	Weight	Temp
	__AM __PM	/				__Pre__Post__Fasting		

Symptoms/Notes:

Date	Time	Blood Pressure	Heart Rate	Resp Rate	Oxygen Level	Blood Sugar (Pre/Post/Fasting)	Weight	Temp
	__AM __PM	/				__Pre__Post__Fasting		

Symptoms/Notes:

Date	Time	Blood Pressure	Heart Rate	Resp Rate	Oxygen Level	Blood Sugar (Pre/Post/Fasting)	Weight	Temp
	__AM __PM	/				__Pre__Post__Fasting		

Symptoms/Notes:

Date	Time	Blood Pressure	Heart Rate	Resp Rate	Oxygen Level	Blood Sugar (Pre/Post/Fasting)	Weight	Temp
	__AM __PM	/				__Pre__Post__Fasting		

Symptoms/Notes:

Date	Time	Blood Pressure	Heart Rate	Resp Rate	Oxygen Level	Blood Sugar (Pre/Post/Fasting)	Weight	Temp
	__AM __PM	/				__Pre__Post__Fasting		

Symptoms/Notes:

Date	Time	Blood Pressure	Heart Rate	Resp Rate	Oxygen Level	Blood Sugar (Pre/Post/Fasting)	Weight	Temp
	__AM __PM	/				__Pre__Post__Fasting		

Symptoms/Notes:

Date	Time	Blood Pressure	Heart Rate	Resp Rate	Oxygen Level	Blood Sugar (Pre/Post/Fasting)	Weight	Temp
	__AM __PM	/				__Pre__Post__Fasting		

Symptoms/Notes:

Date	Time	Blood Pressure	Heart Rate	Resp Rate	Oxygen Level	Blood Sugar (Pre/Post/Fasting)	Weight	Temp
	__AM __PM	/				__Pre__Post__Fasting		

Symptoms/Notes:

Date	Time	Blood Pressure	Heart Rate	Resp Rate	Oxygen Level	Blood Sugar (Pre/Post/Fasting)	Weight	Temp
	__AM __PM	/				__Pre__Post__Fasting		

Symptoms/Notes:

Date	Time	Blood Pressure	Heart Rate	Resp Rate	Oxygen Level	Blood Sugar (Pre/Post/Fasting)	Weight	Temp
	__AM __PM	/				__Pre__Post__Fasting		

Symptoms/Notes:

Date	Time	Blood Pressure	Heart Rate	Resp Rate	Oxygen Level	Blood Sugar (Pre/Post/Fasting)	Weight	Temp
	__AM __PM	/				__Pre__Post__Fasting		

Symptoms/Notes:

Date	Time	Blood Pressure	Heart Rate	Resp Rate	Oxygen Level	Blood Sugar (Pre/Post/Fasting)	Weight	Temp
	__AM __PM	/				__Pre__Post__Fasting		

Symptoms/Notes:

Date	Time	Blood Pressure	Heart Rate	Resp Rate	Oxygen Level	Blood Sugar (Pre/Post/Fasting)	Weight	Temp
	__AM __PM	/				__Pre__Post__Fasting		

Symptoms/Notes:

Date	Time	Blood Pressure	Heart Rate	Resp Rate	Oxygen Level	Blood Sugar (Pre/Post/Fasting)	Weight	Temp
	__AM __PM	/				__Pre__Post__Fasting		

Symptoms/Notes:

Date	Time	Blood Pressure	Heart Rate	Resp Rate	Oxygen Level	Blood Sugar (Pre/Post/Fasting)	Weight	Temp
	__AM __PM	/				__Pre__Post__Fasting		

Symptoms/Notes:

Date	Time	Blood Pressure	Heart Rate	Resp Rate	Oxygen Level	Blood Sugar (Pre/Post/Fasting)	Weight	Temp
	__AM __PM	/				__Pre__Post__Fasting		

Symptoms/Notes:

Date	Time	Blood Pressure	Heart Rate	Resp Rate	Oxygen Level	Blood Sugar (Pre/Post/Fasting)	Weight	Temp
	__AM __PM	/				__Pre__Post__Fasting		

Symptoms/Notes:

Date	Time	Blood Pressure	Heart Rate	Resp Rate	Oxygen Level	Blood Sugar (Pre/Post/Fasting)	Weight	Temp
	__AM __PM	/				__Pre__Post__Fasting		

Symptoms/Notes:

Date	Time	Blood Pressure	Heart Rate	Resp Rate	Oxygen Level	Blood Sugar (Pre/Post/Fasting)	Weight	Temp
	__AM __PM	/				__Pre__Post__Fasting		

Symptoms/Notes:

Date	Time	Blood Pressure	Heart Rate	Resp Rate	Oxygen Level	Blood Sugar (Pre/Post/Fasting)	Weight	Temp
	__AM __PM	/				__Pre__Post__Fasting		

Symptoms/Notes:

Date	Time	Blood Pressure	Heart Rate	Resp Rate	Oxygen Level	Blood Sugar (Pre/Post/Fasting)	Weight	Temp
	__AM __PM	/				__Pre__Post__Fasting		

Symptoms/Notes:

Date	Time	Blood Pressure	Heart Rate	Resp Rate	Oxygen Level	Blood Sugar (Pre/Post/Fasting)	Weight	Temp
	__AM __PM	/				__Pre__Post__Fasting		

Symptoms/Notes:

Date	Time	Blood Pressure	Heart Rate	Resp Rate	Oxygen Level	Blood Sugar (Pre/Post/Fasting)	Weight	Temp
	__AM __PM	/				__Pre__Post__Fasting		

Symptoms/Notes:

Date	Time	Blood Pressure	Heart Rate	Resp Rate	Oxygen Level	Blood Sugar (Pre/Post/Fasting)	Weight	Temp
	__AM __PM	/				__Pre__Post__Fasting		

Symptoms/Notes:

Date	Time	Blood Pressure	Heart Rate	Resp Rate	Oxygen Level	Blood Sugar (Pre/Post/Fasting)	Weight	Temp
	__AM __PM	/				__Pre__Post__Fasting		

Symptoms/Notes:

Date	Time	Blood Pressure	Heart Rate	Resp Rate	Oxygen Level	Blood Sugar (Pre/Post/Fasting)	Weight	Temp
	__AM __PM	/				__Pre__Post__Fasting		

Symptoms/Notes:

Date	Time	Blood Pressure	Heart Rate	Resp Rate	Oxygen Level	Blood Sugar (Pre/Post/Fasting)	Weight	Temp
	__AM __PM	/				__Pre__Post__Fasting		

Symptoms/Notes:

Date	Time	Blood Pressure	Heart Rate	Resp Rate	Oxygen Level	Blood Sugar (Pre/Post/Fasting)	Weight	Temp
	__AM __PM	/				__Pre__Post__Fasting		

Symptoms/Notes:

Date	Time	Blood Pressure	Heart Rate	Resp Rate	Oxygen Level	Blood Sugar (Pre/Post/Fasting)	Weight	Temp
	__AM __PM	/				__Pre__Post__Fasting		

Symptoms/Notes:

Date	Time	Blood Pressure	Heart Rate	Resp Rate	Oxygen Level	Blood Sugar (Pre/Post/Fasting)	Weight	Temp
	__AM __PM	/				__Pre__Post__Fasting		

Symptoms/Notes:

Date	Time	Blood Pressure	Heart Rate	Resp Rate	Oxygen Level	Blood Sugar (Pre/Post/Fasting)	Weight	Temp
	__AM __PM	/				__Pre__Post__Fasting		

Symptoms/Notes:

Date	Time	Blood Pressure	Heart Rate	Resp Rate	Oxygen Level	Blood Sugar (Pre/Post/Fasting)	Weight	Temp
	__AM __PM	/				__Pre__Post__Fasting		

Symptoms/Notes:

Date	Time	Blood Pressure	Heart Rate	Resp Rate	Oxygen Level	Blood Sugar (Pre/Post/Fasting)	Weight	Temp
	__AM __PM	/				__Pre__Post__Fasting		

Symptoms/Notes:

Date	Time	Blood Pressure	Heart Rate	Resp Rate	Oxygen Level	Blood Sugar (Pre/Post/Fasting)	Weight	Temp
	__AM __PM	/				__Pre__Post__Fasting		

Symptoms/Notes:

Date	Time	Blood Pressure	Heart Rate	Resp Rate	Oxygen Level	Blood Sugar (Pre/Post/Fasting)	Weight	Temp
	__AM __PM	/				__Pre__Post__Fasting		

Symptoms/Notes:

Date	Time	Blood Pressure	Heart Rate	Resp Rate	Oxygen Level	Blood Sugar (Pre/Post/Fasting)	Weight	Temp
	__AM __PM	/				__Pre__Post__Fasting		

Symptoms/Notes:

Date	Time	Blood Pressure	Heart Rate	Resp Rate	Oxygen Level	Blood Sugar (Pre/Post/Fasting)	Weight	Temp
	__AM __PM	/				__Pre__Post__Fasting		

Symptoms/Notes:

Date	Time	Blood Pressure	Heart Rate	Resp Rate	Oxygen Level	Blood Sugar (Pre/Post/Fasting)	Weight	Temp
	__AM __PM	/				__Pre__Post__Fasting		

Symptoms/Notes:

Date	Time	Blood Pressure	Heart Rate	Resp Rate	Oxygen Level	Blood Sugar (Pre/Post/Fasting)	Weight	Temp
	__AM __PM	/				__Pre__Post__Fasting		

Symptoms/Notes:

Date	Time	Blood Pressure	Heart Rate	Resp Rate	Oxygen Level	Blood Sugar (Pre/Post/Fasting)	Weight	Temp
	__AM __PM	/				__Pre__Post__Fasting		

Symptoms/Notes:

Date	Time	Blood Pressure	Heart Rate	Resp Rate	Oxygen Level	Blood Sugar (Pre/Post/Fasting)	Weight	Temp
	__AM __PM	/				__Pre__Post__Fasting		

Symptoms/Notes:

Date	Time	Blood Pressure	Heart Rate	Resp Rate	Oxygen Level	Blood Sugar (Pre/Post/Fasting)	Weight	Temp
	__AM __PM	/				__Pre__Post__Fasting		

Symptoms/Notes:

Date	Time	Blood Pressure	Heart Rate	Resp Rate	Oxygen Level	Blood Sugar (Pre/Post/Fasting)	Weight	Temp
	__AM __PM	/				__Pre__Post__Fasting		

Symptoms/Notes:

Date	Time	Blood Pressure	Heart Rate	Resp Rate	Oxygen Level	Blood Sugar (Pre/Post/Fasting)	Weight	Temp
	__AM __PM	/				__Pre__Post__Fasting		

Symptoms/Notes:

Date	Time	Blood Pressure	Heart Rate	Resp Rate	Oxygen Level	Blood Sugar (Pre/Post/Fasting)	Weight	Temp
	__AM __PM	/				__Pre__Post__Fasting		

Symptoms/Notes:

Date	Time	Blood Pressure	Heart Rate	Resp Rate	Oxygen Level	Blood Sugar (Pre/Post/Fasting)	Weight	Temp
	__AM __PM	/				__Pre__Post__Fasting		

Symptoms/Notes:

Date	Time	Blood Pressure	Heart Rate	Resp Rate	Oxygen Level	Blood Sugar (Pre/Post/Fasting)	Weight	Temp
	__AM __PM	/				__Pre__Post__Fasting		

Symptoms/Notes:

Date	Time	Blood Pressure	Heart Rate	Resp Rate	Oxygen Level	Blood Sugar (Pre/Post/Fasting)	Weight	Temp
	__AM __PM	/				__Pre__Post__Fasting		

Symptoms/Notes:

Date	Time	Blood Pressure	Heart Rate	Resp Rate	Oxygen Level	Blood Sugar (Pre/Post/Fasting)	Weight	Temp
	__AM __PM	/				__Pre__Post__Fasting		

Symptoms/Notes:

Date	Time	Blood Pressure	Heart Rate	Resp Rate	Oxygen Level	Blood Sugar (Pre/Post/Fasting)	Weight	Temp
	__AM __PM	/				__Pre__Post__Fasting		

Symptoms/Notes:

Date	Time	Blood Pressure	Heart Rate	Resp Rate	Oxygen Level	Blood Sugar (Pre/Post/Fasting)	Weight	Temp
	__AM __PM	/				__Pre__Post__Fasting		

Symptoms/Notes:

Date	Time	Blood Pressure	Heart Rate	Resp Rate	Oxygen Level	Blood Sugar (Pre/Post/Fasting)	Weight	Temp
	__AM __PM	/				__Pre__Post__Fasting		

Symptoms/Notes:

Date	Time	Blood Pressure	Heart Rate	Resp Rate	Oxygen Level	Blood Sugar (Pre/Post/Fasting)	Weight	Temp
	__AM __PM	/				__Pre__Post__Fasting		

Symptoms/Notes:

Date	Time	Blood Pressure	Heart Rate	Resp Rate	Oxygen Level	Blood Sugar (Pre/Post/Fasting)	Weight	Temp
	__AM __PM	/				__Pre__Post__Fasting		

Symptoms/Notes:

Date	Time	Blood Pressure	Heart Rate	Resp Rate	Oxygen Level	Blood Sugar (Pre/Post/Fasting)	Weight	Temp
	__AM __PM	/				__Pre__Post__Fasting		

Symptoms/Notes:

Date	Time	Blood Pressure	Heart Rate	Resp Rate	Oxygen Level	Blood Sugar (Pre/Post/Fasting)	Weight	Temp
	__AM __PM	/				__Pre__Post__Fasting		

Symptoms/Notes:

Date	Time	Blood Pressure	Heart Rate	Resp Rate	Oxygen Level	Blood Sugar (Pre/Post/Fasting)	Weight	Temp
	__AM __PM	/				__Pre__Post__Fasting		

Symptoms/Notes:

Date	Time	Blood Pressure	Heart Rate	Resp Rate	Oxygen Level	Blood Sugar (Pre/Post/Fasting)	Weight	Temp
	__AM __PM	/				__Pre__Post__Fasting		

Symptoms/Notes:

Date	Time	Blood Pressure	Heart Rate	Resp Rate	Oxygen Level	Blood Sugar (Pre/Post/Fasting)	Weight	Temp
	__AM __PM	/				__Pre__Post__Fasting		

Symptoms/Notes:

Date	Time	Blood Pressure	Heart Rate	Resp Rate	Oxygen Level	Blood Sugar (Pre/Post/Fasting)	Weight	Temp
	__AM __PM	/				__Pre__Post__Fasting		

Symptoms/Notes:

Date	Time	Blood Pressure	Heart Rate	Resp Rate	Oxygen Level	Blood Sugar (Pre/Post/Fasting)	Weight	Temp
	__AM __PM	/				__Pre__Post__Fasting		

Symptoms/Notes:

Date	Time	Blood Pressure	Heart Rate	Resp Rate	Oxygen Level	Blood Sugar (Pre/Post/Fasting)	Weight	Temp
	__AM __PM	/				__Pre__Post__Fasting		

Symptoms/Notes:

Date	Time	Blood Pressure	Heart Rate	Resp Rate	Oxygen Level	Blood Sugar (Pre/Post/Fasting)	Weight	Temp
	__AM __PM	/				__Pre__Post__Fasting		

Symptoms/Notes:

Date	Time	Blood Pressure	Heart Rate	Resp Rate	Oxygen Level	Blood Sugar (Pre/Post/Fasting)	Weight	Temp
	__AM __PM	/				__Pre__Post__Fasting		

Symptoms/Notes:

Date	Time	Blood Pressure	Heart Rate	Resp Rate	Oxygen Level	Blood Sugar (Pre/Post/Fasting)	Weight	Temp
	__AM __PM	/				__Pre__Post__Fasting		

Symptoms/Notes:

Date	Time	Blood Pressure	Heart Rate	Resp Rate	Oxygen Level	Blood Sugar (Pre/Post/Fasting)	Weight	Temp
	__AM __PM	/				__Pre__Post__Fasting		

Symptoms/Notes:

Date	Time	Blood Pressure	Heart Rate	Resp Rate	Oxygen Level	Blood Sugar (Pre/Post/Fasting)	Weight	Temp
	__AM __PM	/				__Pre__Post__Fasting		

Symptoms/Notes:

Date	Time	Blood Pressure	Heart Rate	Resp Rate	Oxygen Level	Blood Sugar (Pre/Post/Fasting)	Weight	Temp
	__AM __PM	/				__Pre__Post__Fasting		

Symptoms/Notes:

Date	Time	Blood Pressure	Heart Rate	Resp Rate	Oxygen Level	Blood Sugar (Pre/Post/Fasting)	Weight	Temp
	__AM __PM	/				__Pre__Post__Fasting		

Symptoms/Notes:

Date	Time	Blood Pressure	Heart Rate	Resp Rate	Oxygen Level	Blood Sugar (Pre/Post/Fasting)	Weight	Temp
	__AM __PM	/				__Pre__Post__Fasting		

Symptoms/Notes:

Date	Time	Blood Pressure	Heart Rate	Resp Rate	Oxygen Level	Blood Sugar (Pre/Post/Fasting)	Weight	Temp
	__AM __PM	/				__Pre__Post__Fasting		

Symptoms/Notes:

Date	Time	Blood Pressure	Heart Rate	Resp Rate	Oxygen Level	Blood Sugar (Pre/Post/Fasting)	Weight	Temp
	__AM __PM	/				__Pre__Post__Fasting		

Symptoms/Notes:

Date	Time	Blood Pressure	Heart Rate	Resp Rate	Oxygen Level	Blood Sugar (Pre/Post/Fasting)	Weight	Temp
	__AM __PM	/				__Pre__Post__Fasting		

Symptoms/Notes:

Date	Time	Blood Pressure	Heart Rate	Resp Rate	Oxygen Level	Blood Sugar (Pre/Post/Fasting)	Weight	Temp
	__AM __PM	/				__Pre__Post__Fasting		

Symptoms/Notes:

Date	Time	Blood Pressure	Heart Rate	Resp Rate	Oxygen Level	Blood Sugar (Pre/Post/Fasting)	Weight	Temp
	__AM __PM	/				__Pre__Post__Fasting		

Symptoms/Notes:

Date	Time	Blood Pressure	Heart Rate	Resp Rate	Oxygen Level	Blood Sugar (Pre/Post/Fasting)	Weight	Temp
	__AM __PM	/				__Pre__Post__Fasting		

Symptoms/Notes:

Date	Time	Blood Pressure	Heart Rate	Resp Rate	Oxygen Level	Blood Sugar (Pre/Post/Fasting)	Weight	Temp
	__AM __PM	/				__Pre__Post__Fasting		

Symptoms/Notes:

Date	Time	Blood Pressure	Heart Rate	Resp Rate	Oxygen Level	Blood Sugar (Pre/Post/Fasting)	Weight	Temp
	__AM __PM	/				__Pre__Post__Fasting		

Symptoms/Notes:

Date	Time	Blood Pressure	Heart Rate	Resp Rate	Oxygen Level	Blood Sugar (Pre/Post/Fasting)	Weight	Temp
	__AM __PM	/				__Pre__Post__Fasting		

Symptoms/Notes:

Date	Time	Blood Pressure	Heart Rate	Resp Rate	Oxygen Level	Blood Sugar (Pre/Post/Fasting)	Weight	Temp
	__AM __PM	/				__Pre__Post__Fasting		

Symptoms/Notes:

Date	Time	Blood Pressure	Heart Rate	Resp Rate	Oxygen Level	Blood Sugar (Pre/Post/Fasting)	Weight	Temp
	__AM __PM	/				__Pre__Post__Fasting		

Symptoms/Notes:

Date	Time	Blood Pressure	Heart Rate	Resp Rate	Oxygen Level	Blood Sugar (Pre/Post/Fasting)	Weight	Temp
	__AM __PM	/				__Pre__Post__Fasting		

Symptoms/Notes:

Date	Time	Blood Pressure	Heart Rate	Resp Rate	Oxygen Level	Blood Sugar (Pre/Post/Fasting)	Weight	Temp
	__AM __PM	/				__Pre__Post__Fasting		

Symptoms/Notes:

Date	Time	Blood Pressure	Heart Rate	Resp Rate	Oxygen Level	Blood Sugar (Pre/Post/Fasting)	Weight	Temp
	__AM __PM	/				__Pre__Post__Fasting		

Symptoms/Notes:

Date	Time	Blood Pressure	Heart Rate	Resp Rate	Oxygen Level	Blood Sugar (Pre/Post/Fasting)	Weight	Temp
	__AM __PM	/				__Pre__Post__Fasting		

Symptoms/Notes:

Date	Time	Blood Pressure	Heart Rate	Resp Rate	Oxygen Level	Blood Sugar (Pre/Post/Fasting)	Weight	Temp
	__AM __PM	/				__Pre__Post__Fasting		

Symptoms/Notes:

Date	Time	Blood Pressure	Heart Rate	Resp Rate	Oxygen Level	Blood Sugar (Pre/Post/Fasting)	Weight	Temp
	__AM __PM	/				__Pre__Post__Fasting		

Symptoms/Notes:

Date	Time	Blood Pressure	Heart Rate	Resp Rate	Oxygen Level	Blood Sugar (Pre/Post/Fasting)	Weight	Temp
	__AM __PM	/				__Pre__Post__Fasting		

Symptoms/Notes:

Date	Time	Blood Pressure	Heart Rate	Resp Rate	Oxygen Level	Blood Sugar (Pre/Post/Fasting)	Weight	Temp
	__AM __PM	/				__Pre__Post__Fasting		

Symptoms/Notes:

Date	Time	Blood Pressure	Heart Rate	Resp Rate	Oxygen Level	Blood Sugar (Pre/Post/Fasting)	Weight	Temp
	__AM __PM	/				__Pre__Post__Fasting		

Symptoms/Notes:

Date	Time	Blood Pressure	Heart Rate	Resp Rate	Oxygen Level	Blood Sugar (Pre/Post/Fasting)	Weight	Temp
	__AM __PM	/				__Pre__Post__Fasting		

Symptoms/Notes:

Date	Time	Blood Pressure	Heart Rate	Resp Rate	Oxygen Level	Blood Sugar (Pre/Post/Fasting)	Weight	Temp
	__AM __PM	/				__Pre__Post__Fasting		

Symptoms/Notes:

Date	Time	Blood Pressure	Heart Rate	Resp Rate	Oxygen Level	Blood Sugar (Pre/Post/Fasting)	Weight	Temp
	__AM __PM	/				__Pre__Post__Fasting		

Symptoms/Notes:

Date	Time	Blood Pressure	Heart Rate	Resp Rate	Oxygen Level	Blood Sugar (Pre/Post/Fasting)	Weight	Temp
	__AM __PM	/				__Pre__Post__Fasting		

Symptoms/Notes:

Date	Time	Blood Pressure	Heart Rate	Resp Rate	Oxygen Level	Blood Sugar (Pre/Post/Fasting)	Weight	Temp
	__AM __PM	/				__Pre__Post__Fasting		

Symptoms/Notes:

Date	Time	Blood Pressure	Heart Rate	Resp Rate	Oxygen Level	Blood Sugar (Pre/Post/Fasting)	Weight	Temp
	__AM __PM	/				__Pre__Post__Fasting		

Symptoms/Notes:

Date	Time	Blood Pressure	Heart Rate	Resp Rate	Oxygen Level	Blood Sugar (Pre/Post/Fasting)	Weight	Temp
	__AM __PM	/				__Pre__Post__Fasting		

Symptoms/Notes:

Date	Time	Blood Pressure	Heart Rate	Resp Rate	Oxygen Level	Blood Sugar (Pre/Post/Fasting)	Weight	Temp
	__AM __PM	/				__Pre__Post__Fasting		

Symptoms/Notes:

Date	Time	Blood Pressure	Heart Rate	Resp Rate	Oxygen Level	Blood Sugar (Pre/Post/Fasting)	Weight	Temp
	__AM __PM	/				__Pre__Post__Fasting		

Symptoms/Notes:

Date	Time	Blood Pressure	Heart Rate	Resp Rate	Oxygen Level	Blood Sugar (Pre/Post/Fasting)	Weight	Temp
	__AM __PM	/				__Pre__Post__Fasting		

Symptoms/Notes:

Date	Time	Blood Pressure	Heart Rate	Resp Rate	Oxygen Level	Blood Sugar (Pre/Post/Fasting)	Weight	Temp
	__AM __PM	/				__Pre__Post__Fasting		

Symptoms/Notes:

Date	Time	Blood Pressure	Heart Rate	Resp Rate	Oxygen Level	Blood Sugar (Pre/Post/Fasting)	Weight	Temp
	__AM __PM	/				__Pre__Post__Fasting		

Symptoms/Notes:

Date	Time	Blood Pressure	Heart Rate	Resp Rate	Oxygen Level	Blood Sugar (Pre/Post/Fasting)	Weight	Temp
	__AM __PM	/				__Pre__Post__Fasting		

Symptoms/Notes:

Date	Time	Blood Pressure	Heart Rate	Resp Rate	Oxygen Level	Blood Sugar (Pre/Post/Fasting)	Weight	Temp
	__AM __PM	/				__Pre__Post__Fasting		

Symptoms/Notes:

Date	Time	Blood Pressure	Heart Rate	Resp Rate	Oxygen Level	Blood Sugar (Pre/Post/Fasting)	Weight	Temp
	__AM __PM	/				__Pre__Post__Fasting		

Symptoms/Notes:

Date	Time	Blood Pressure	Heart Rate	Resp Rate	Oxygen Level	Blood Sugar (Pre/Post/Fasting)	Weight	Temp
	__AM __PM	/				__Pre__Post__Fasting		

Symptoms/Notes:

Date	Time	Blood Pressure	Heart Rate	Resp Rate	Oxygen Level	Blood Sugar (Pre/Post/Fasting)	Weight	Temp
	__AM __PM	/				__Pre__Post__Fasting		

Symptoms/Notes:

Date	Time	Blood Pressure	Heart Rate	Resp Rate	Oxygen Level	Blood Sugar (Pre/Post/Fasting)	Weight	Temp
	__AM __PM	/				__Pre__Post__Fasting		

Symptoms/Notes:

Date	Time	Blood Pressure	Heart Rate	Resp Rate	Oxygen Level	Blood Sugar (Pre/Post/Fasting)	Weight	Temp
	__AM __PM	/				__Pre__Post__Fasting		

Symptoms/Notes:

Date	Time	Blood Pressure	Heart Rate	Resp Rate	Oxygen Level	Blood Sugar (Pre/Post/Fasting)	Weight	Temp
	__AM __PM	/				__Pre__Post__Fasting		

Symptoms/Notes:

Date	Time	Blood Pressure	Heart Rate	Resp Rate	Oxygen Level	Blood Sugar (Pre/Post/Fasting)	Weight	Temp
	__AM __PM	/				__Pre__Post__Fasting		

Symptoms/Notes:

Date	Time	Blood Pressure	Heart Rate	Resp Rate	Oxygen Level	Blood Sugar (Pre/Post/Fasting)	Weight	Temp
	__AM __PM	/				__Pre__Post__Fasting		

Symptoms/Notes:

Date	Time	Blood Pressure	Heart Rate	Resp Rate	Oxygen Level	Blood Sugar (Pre/Post/Fasting)	Weight	Temp
	__AM __PM	/				__Pre__Post__Fasting		

Symptoms/Notes:

Date	Time	Blood Pressure	Heart Rate	Resp Rate	Oxygen Level	Blood Sugar (Pre/Post/Fasting)	Weight	Temp
	__AM __PM	/				__Pre__Post__Fasting		

Symptoms/Notes:

Date	Time	Blood Pressure	Heart Rate	Resp Rate	Oxygen Level	Blood Sugar (Pre/Post/Fasting)	Weight	Temp
	__AM __PM	/				__Pre__Post__Fasting		

Symptoms/Notes:

Date	Time	Blood Pressure	Heart Rate	Resp Rate	Oxygen Level	Blood Sugar (Pre/Post/Fasting)	Weight	Temp
	__AM __PM	/				__Pre__Post__Fasting		

Symptoms/Notes:

Date	Time	Blood Pressure	Heart Rate	Resp Rate	Oxygen Level	Blood Sugar (Pre/Post/Fasting)	Weight	Temp
	__AM __PM	/				__Pre__Post__Fasting		

Symptoms/Notes:

Date	Time	Blood Pressure	Heart Rate	Resp Rate	Oxygen Level	Blood Sugar (Pre/Post/Fasting)	Weight	Temp
	__AM __PM	/				__Pre__Post__Fasting		

Symptoms/Notes:

Date	Time	Blood Pressure	Heart Rate	Resp Rate	Oxygen Level	Blood Sugar (Pre/Post/Fasting)	Weight	Temp
	__AM __PM	/				__Pre__Post__Fasting		

Symptoms/Notes:

Date	Time	Blood Pressure	Heart Rate	Resp Rate	Oxygen Level	Blood Sugar (Pre/Post/Fasting)	Weight	Temp
	__AM __PM	/				__Pre__Post__Fasting		

Symptoms/Notes:

Date	Time	Blood Pressure	Heart Rate	Resp Rate	Oxygen Level	Blood Sugar (Pre/Post/Fasting)	Weight	Temp
	__AM __PM	/				__Pre__Post__Fasting		

Symptoms/Notes:

Date	Time	Blood Pressure	Heart Rate	Resp Rate	Oxygen Level	Blood Sugar (Pre/Post/Fasting)	Weight	Temp
	__AM __PM	/				__Pre__Post__Fasting		

Symptoms/Notes:

Date	Time	Blood Pressure	Heart Rate	Resp Rate	Oxygen Level	Blood Sugar (Pre/Post/Fasting)	Weight	Temp
	__AM __PM	/				__Pre__Post__Fasting		

Symptoms/Notes:

Date	Time	Blood Pressure	Heart Rate	Resp Rate	Oxygen Level	Blood Sugar (Pre/Post/Fasting)	Weight	Temp
	__AM __PM	/				__Pre__Post__Fasting		

Symptoms/Notes:

Date	Time	Blood Pressure	Heart Rate	Resp Rate	Oxygen Level	Blood Sugar (Pre/Post/Fasting)	Weight	Temp
	__AM __PM	/				__Pre__Post__Fasting		

Symptoms/Notes:

Date	Time	Blood Pressure	Heart Rate	Resp Rate	Oxygen Level	Blood Sugar (Pre/Post/Fasting)	Weight	Temp
	__AM __PM	/				__Pre__Post__Fasting		

Symptoms/Notes:

Date	Time	Blood Pressure	Heart Rate	Resp Rate	Oxygen Level	Blood Sugar (Pre/Post/Fasting)	Weight	Temp
	__AM __PM	/				__Pre__Post__Fasting		

Symptoms/Notes:

Date	Time	Blood Pressure	Heart Rate	Resp Rate	Oxygen Level	Blood Sugar (Pre/Post/Fasting)	Weight	Temp
	__AM __PM	/				__Pre__Post__Fasting		

Symptoms/Notes:

Date	Time	Blood Pressure	Heart Rate	Resp Rate	Oxygen Level	Blood Sugar (Pre/Post/Fasting)	Weight	Temp
	__AM __PM	/				__Pre__Post__Fasting		

Symptoms/Notes:

Date	Time	Blood Pressure	Heart Rate	Resp Rate	Oxygen Level	Blood Sugar (Pre/Post/Fasting)	Weight	Temp
	__AM __PM	/				__Pre__Post__Fasting		

Symptoms/Notes:

Date	Time	Blood Pressure	Heart Rate	Resp Rate	Oxygen Level	Blood Sugar (Pre/Post/Fasting)	Weight	Temp
	__AM __PM	/				__Pre__Post__Fasting		

Symptoms/Notes:

Date	Time	Blood Pressure	Heart Rate	Resp Rate	Oxygen Level	Blood Sugar (Pre/Post/Fasting)	Weight	Temp
	__AM __PM	/				__Pre__Post__Fasting		

Symptoms/Notes:

Date	Time	Blood Pressure	Heart Rate	Resp Rate	Oxygen Level	Blood Sugar (Pre/Post/Fasting)	Weight	Temp
	__AM __PM	/				__Pre__Post__Fasting		

Symptoms/Notes:

Date	Time	Blood Pressure	Heart Rate	Resp Rate	Oxygen Level	Blood Sugar (Pre/Post/Fasting)	Weight	Temp
	__AM __PM	/				__Pre__Post__Fasting		

Symptoms/Notes:

Date	Time	Blood Pressure	Heart Rate	Resp Rate	Oxygen Level	Blood Sugar (Pre/Post/Fasting)	Weight	Temp
	__AM __PM	/				__Pre__Post__Fasting		

Symptoms/Notes:

Date	Time	Blood Pressure	Heart Rate	Resp Rate	Oxygen Level	Blood Sugar (Pre/Post/Fasting)	Weight	Temp
	__AM __PM	/				__Pre__Post__Fasting		

Symptoms/Notes:

Date	Time	Blood Pressure	Heart Rate	Resp Rate	Oxygen Level	Blood Sugar (Pre/Post/Fasting)	Weight	Temp
	__AM __PM	/				__Pre__Post__Fasting		

Symptoms/Notes:

Date	Time	Blood Pressure	Heart Rate	Resp Rate	Oxygen Level	Blood Sugar (Pre/Post/Fasting)	Weight	Temp
	__AM __PM	/				__Pre__Post__Fasting		

Symptoms/Notes:

Date	Time	Blood Pressure	Heart Rate	Resp Rate	Oxygen Level	Blood Sugar (Pre/Post/Fasting)	Weight	Temp
	__AM __PM	/				__Pre__Post__Fasting		

Symptoms/Notes:

Date	Time	Blood Pressure	Heart Rate	Resp Rate	Oxygen Level	Blood Sugar (Pre/Post/Fasting)	Weight	Temp
	__AM __PM	/				__Pre__Post__Fasting		

Symptoms/Notes:

Date	Time	Blood Pressure	Heart Rate	Resp Rate	Oxygen Level	Blood Sugar (Pre/Post/Fasting)	Weight	Temp
	__AM __PM	/				__Pre__Post__Fasting		

Symptoms/Notes:

Date	Time	Blood Pressure	Heart Rate	Resp Rate	Oxygen Level	Blood Sugar (Pre/Post/Fasting)	Weight	Temp
	__AM __PM	/				__Pre__Post__Fasting		

Symptoms/Notes:

Date	Time	Blood Pressure	Heart Rate	Resp Rate	Oxygen Level	Blood Sugar (Pre/Post/Fasting)	Weight	Temp
	__AM __PM	/				__Pre__Post__Fasting		

Symptoms/Notes:

Date	Time	Blood Pressure	Heart Rate	Resp Rate	Oxygen Level	Blood Sugar (Pre/Post/Fasting)	Weight	Temp
	__AM __PM	/				__Pre__Post__Fasting		

Symptoms/Notes:

Date	Time	Blood Pressure	Heart Rate	Resp Rate	Oxygen Level	Blood Sugar (Pre/Post/Fasting)	Weight	Temp
	__AM __PM	/				__Pre__Post__Fasting		

Symptoms/Notes:

Date	Time	Blood Pressure	Heart Rate	Resp Rate	Oxygen Level	Blood Sugar (Pre/Post/Fasting)	Weight	Temp
	__AM __PM	/				__Pre__Post__Fasting		

Symptoms/Notes:

Date	Time	Blood Pressure	Heart Rate	Resp Rate	Oxygen Level	Blood Sugar (Pre/Post/Fasting)	Weight	Temp
	__AM __PM	/				__Pre__Post__Fasting		

Symptoms/Notes:

Date	Time	Blood Pressure	Heart Rate	Resp Rate	Oxygen Level	Blood Sugar (Pre/Post/Fasting)	Weight	Temp
	__AM __PM	/				__Pre__Post__Fasting		

Symptoms/Notes:

Date	Time	Blood Pressure	Heart Rate	Resp Rate	Oxygen Level	Blood Sugar (Pre/Post/Fasting)	Weight	Temp
	__AM __PM	/				__Pre__Post__Fasting		

Symptoms/Notes:

Date	Time	Blood Pressure	Heart Rate	Resp Rate	Oxygen Level	Blood Sugar (Pre/Post/Fasting)	Weight	Temp
	__AM __PM	/				__Pre__Post__Fasting		

Symptoms/Notes:

Date	Time	Blood Pressure	Heart Rate	Resp Rate	Oxygen Level	Blood Sugar (Pre/Post/Fasting)	Weight	Temp
	__AM __PM	/				__Pre__Post__Fasting		

Symptoms/Notes:

Date	Time	Blood Pressure	Heart Rate	Resp Rate	Oxygen Level	Blood Sugar (Pre/Post/Fasting)	Weight	Temp
	__AM __PM	/				__Pre__Post__Fasting		

Symptoms/Notes:

Date	Time	Blood Pressure	Heart Rate	Resp Rate	Oxygen Level	Blood Sugar (Pre/Post/Fasting)	Weight	Temp
	__AM __PM	/				__Pre__Post__Fasting		

Symptoms/Notes:

Date	Time	Blood Pressure	Heart Rate	Resp Rate	Oxygen Level	Blood Sugar (Pre/Post/Fasting)	Weight	Temp
	__AM __PM	/				__Pre__Post__Fasting		

Symptoms/Notes:

Date	Time	Blood Pressure	Heart Rate	Resp Rate	Oxygen Level	Blood Sugar (Pre/Post/Fasting)	Weight	Temp
	__AM __PM	/				__Pre__Post__Fasting		

Symptoms/Notes:

Date	Time	Blood Pressure	Heart Rate	Resp Rate	Oxygen Level	Blood Sugar (Pre/Post/Fasting)	Weight	Temp
	__AM __PM	/				__Pre__Post__Fasting		

Symptoms/Notes:

Date	Time	Blood Pressure	Heart Rate	Resp Rate	Oxygen Level	Blood Sugar (Pre/Post/Fasting)	Weight	Temp
	__AM __PM	/				__Pre__Post__Fasting		

Symptoms/Notes:

Date	Time	Blood Pressure	Heart Rate	Resp Rate	Oxygen Level	Blood Sugar (Pre/Post/Fasting)	Weight	Temp
	__AM __PM	/				__Pre__Post__Fasting		

Symptoms/Notes:

Date	Time	Blood Pressure	Heart Rate	Resp Rate	Oxygen Level	Blood Sugar (Pre/Post/Fasting)	Weight	Temp
	__AM __PM	/				__Pre__Post__Fasting		

Symptoms/Notes:

Date	Time	Blood Pressure	Heart Rate	Resp Rate	Oxygen Level	Blood Sugar (Pre/Post/Fasting)	Weight	Temp
	__AM __PM	/				__Pre__Post__Fasting		

Symptoms/Notes:

Date	Time	Blood Pressure	Heart Rate	Resp Rate	Oxygen Level	Blood Sugar (Pre/Post/Fasting)	Weight	Temp
	__AM __PM	/				__Pre__Post__Fasting		

Symptoms/Notes:

Date	Time	Blood Pressure	Heart Rate	Resp Rate	Oxygen Level	Blood Sugar (Pre/Post/Fasting)	Weight	Temp
	__AM __PM	/				__Pre__Post__Fasting		

Symptoms/Notes:

Date	Time	Blood Pressure	Heart Rate	Resp Rate	Oxygen Level	Blood Sugar (Pre/Post/Fasting)	Weight	Temp
	__AM __PM	/				__Pre__Post__Fasting		

Symptoms/Notes:

Date	Time	Blood Pressure	Heart Rate	Resp Rate	Oxygen Level	Blood Sugar (Pre/Post/Fasting)	Weight	Temp
	__AM __PM	/				__Pre__Post__Fasting		

Symptoms/Notes:

Date	Time	Blood Pressure	Heart Rate	Resp Rate	Oxygen Level	Blood Sugar (Pre/Post/Fasting)	Weight	Temp
	__AM __PM	/				__Pre__Post__Fasting		

Symptoms/Notes:

Date	Time	Blood Pressure	Heart Rate	Resp Rate	Oxygen Level	Blood Sugar (Pre/Post/Fasting)	Weight	Temp
	__AM __PM	/				__Pre__Post__Fasting		

Symptoms/Notes:

Date	Time	Blood Pressure	Heart Rate	Resp Rate	Oxygen Level	Blood Sugar (Pre/Post/Fasting)	Weight	Temp
	__AM __PM	/				__Pre__Post__Fasting		

Symptoms/Notes:

Date	Time	Blood Pressure	Heart Rate	Resp Rate	Oxygen Level	Blood Sugar (Pre/Post/Fasting)	Weight	Temp
	__AM __PM	/				__Pre__Post__Fasting		

Symptoms/Notes:

Date	Time	Blood Pressure	Heart Rate	Resp Rate	Oxygen Level	Blood Sugar (Pre/Post/Fasting)	Weight	Temp
	__AM __PM	/				__Pre__Post__Fasting		

Symptoms/Notes:

Date	Time	Blood Pressure	Heart Rate	Resp Rate	Oxygen Level	Blood Sugar (Pre/Post/Fasting)	Weight	Temp
	__AM __PM	/				__Pre__Post__Fasting		

Symptoms/Notes:

Date	Time	Blood Pressure	Heart Rate	Resp Rate	Oxygen Level	Blood Sugar (Pre/Post/Fasting)	Weight	Temp
	__AM __PM	/				__Pre__Post__Fasting		

Symptoms/Notes:

Date	Time	Blood Pressure	Heart Rate	Resp Rate	Oxygen Level	Blood Sugar (Pre/Post/Fasting)	Weight	Temp
	__AM __PM	/				__Pre__Post__Fasting		

Symptoms/Notes:

Date	Time	Blood Pressure	Heart Rate	Resp Rate	Oxygen Level	Blood Sugar (Pre/Post/Fasting)	Weight	Temp
	__AM __PM	/				__Pre__Post__Fasting		

Symptoms/Notes:

Date	Time	Blood Pressure	Heart Rate	Resp Rate	Oxygen Level	Blood Sugar (Pre/Post/Fasting)	Weight	Temp
	__AM __PM	/				__Pre__Post__Fasting		

Symptoms/Notes:

Date	Time	Blood Pressure	Heart Rate	Resp Rate	Oxygen Level	Blood Sugar (Pre/Post/Fasting)	Weight	Temp
	__AM __PM	/				__Pre__Post__Fasting		

Symptoms/Notes:

Date	Time	Blood Pressure	Heart Rate	Resp Rate	Oxygen Level	Blood Sugar (Pre/Post/Fasting)	Weight	Temp
	__AM __PM	/				__Pre__Post__Fasting		

Symptoms/Notes:

Date	Time	Blood Pressure	Heart Rate	Resp Rate	Oxygen Level	Blood Sugar (Pre/Post/Fasting)	Weight	Temp
	__AM __PM	/				__Pre__Post__Fasting		

Symptoms/Notes:

Date	Time	Blood Pressure	Heart Rate	Resp Rate	Oxygen Level	Blood Sugar (Pre/Post/Fasting)	Weight	Temp
	__AM __PM	/				__Pre__Post__Fasting		

Symptoms/Notes:

Date	Time	Blood Pressure	Heart Rate	Resp Rate	Oxygen Level	Blood Sugar (Pre/Post/Fasting)	Weight	Temp
	__AM __PM	/				__Pre__Post__Fasting		

Symptoms/Notes:

Date	Time	Blood Pressure	Heart Rate	Resp Rate	Oxygen Level	Blood Sugar (Pre/Post/Fasting)	Weight	Temp
	__AM __PM	/				__Pre__Post__Fasting		

Symptoms/Notes:

Date	Time	Blood Pressure	Heart Rate	Resp Rate	Oxygen Level	Blood Sugar (Pre/Post/Fasting)	Weight	Temp
	__AM __PM	/				__Pre__Post__Fasting		

Symptoms/Notes:

Date	Time	Blood Pressure	Heart Rate	Resp Rate	Oxygen Level	Blood Sugar (Pre/Post/Fasting)	Weight	Temp
	__AM __PM	/				__Pre__Post__Fasting		

Symptoms/Notes:

Date	Time	Blood Pressure	Heart Rate	Resp Rate	Oxygen Level	Blood Sugar (Pre/Post/Fasting)	Weight	Temp
	__AM __PM	/				__Pre__Post__Fasting		

Symptoms/Notes:

Date	Time	Blood Pressure	Heart Rate	Resp Rate	Oxygen Level	Blood Sugar (Pre/Post/Fasting)	Weight	Temp
	__AM __PM	/				__Pre__Post__Fasting		

Symptoms/Notes:

Date	Time	Blood Pressure	Heart Rate	Resp Rate	Oxygen Level	Blood Sugar (Pre/Post/Fasting)	Weight	Temp
	__AM __PM	/				__Pre__Post__Fasting		

Symptoms/Notes:

Date	Time	Blood Pressure	Heart Rate	Resp Rate	Oxygen Level	Blood Sugar (Pre/Post/Fasting)	Weight	Temp
	__AM __PM	/				__Pre__Post__Fasting		

Symptoms/Notes:

Date	Time	Blood Pressure	Heart Rate	Resp Rate	Oxygen Level	Blood Sugar (Pre/Post/Fasting)	Weight	Temp
	__AM __PM	/				__Pre__Post__Fasting		

Symptoms/Notes:

Date	Time	Blood Pressure	Heart Rate	Resp Rate	Oxygen Level	Blood Sugar (Pre/Post/Fasting)	Weight	Temp
	__AM __PM	/				__Pre__Post__Fasting		

Symptoms/Notes:

Date	Time	Blood Pressure	Heart Rate	Resp Rate	Oxygen Level	Blood Sugar (Pre/Post/Fasting)	Weight	Temp
	__AM __PM	/				__Pre__Post__Fasting		

Symptoms/Notes:

Date	Time	Blood Pressure	Heart Rate	Resp Rate	Oxygen Level	Blood Sugar (Pre/Post/Fasting)	Weight	Temp
	__AM __PM	/				__Pre__Post__Fasting		

Symptoms/Notes:

Date	Time	Blood Pressure	Heart Rate	Resp Rate	Oxygen Level	Blood Sugar (Pre/Post/Fasting)	Weight	Temp
	__AM __PM	/				__Pre__Post__Fasting		

Symptoms/Notes:

Date	Time	Blood Pressure	Heart Rate	Resp Rate	Oxygen Level	Blood Sugar (Pre/Post/Fasting)	Weight	Temp
	__AM __PM	/				__Pre__Post__Fasting		

Symptoms/Notes:

Date	Time	Blood Pressure	Heart Rate	Resp Rate	Oxygen Level	Blood Sugar (Pre/Post/Fasting)	Weight	Temp
	__AM __PM	/				__Pre__Post__Fasting		

Symptoms/Notes:

Date	Time	Blood Pressure	Heart Rate	Resp Rate	Oxygen Level	Blood Sugar (Pre/Post/Fasting)	Weight	Temp
	__AM __PM	/				__Pre__Post__Fasting		

Symptoms/Notes:

Date	Time	Blood Pressure	Heart Rate	Resp Rate	Oxygen Level	Blood Sugar (Pre/Post/Fasting)	Weight	Temp
	__AM __PM	/				__Pre__Post__Fasting		

Symptoms/Notes:

Date	Time	Blood Pressure	Heart Rate	Resp Rate	Oxygen Level	Blood Sugar (Pre/Post/Fasting)	Weight	Temp
	__AM __PM	/				__Pre__Post__Fasting		

Symptoms/Notes:

Date	Time	Blood Pressure	Heart Rate	Resp Rate	Oxygen Level	Blood Sugar (Pre/Post/Fasting)	Weight	Temp
	__AM __PM	/				__Pre__Post__Fasting		

Symptoms/Notes:

Date	Time	Blood Pressure	Heart Rate	Resp Rate	Oxygen Level	Blood Sugar (Pre/Post/Fasting)	Weight	Temp
	__AM __PM	/				__Pre__Post__Fasting		

Symptoms/Notes:

Date	Time	Blood Pressure	Heart Rate	Resp Rate	Oxygen Level	Blood Sugar (Pre/Post/Fasting)	Weight	Temp
	__AM __PM	/				__Pre__Post__Fasting		

Symptoms/Notes:

Date	Time	Blood Pressure	Heart Rate	Resp Rate	Oxygen Level	Blood Sugar (Pre/Post/Fasting)	Weight	Temp
	__AM __PM	/				__Pre__Post__Fasting		

Symptoms/Notes:

Date	Time	Blood Pressure	Heart Rate	Resp Rate	Oxygen Level	Blood Sugar (Pre/Post/Fasting)	Weight	Temp
	__AM __PM	/				__Pre__Post__Fasting		

Symptoms/Notes:

Date	Time	Blood Pressure	Heart Rate	Resp Rate	Oxygen Level	Blood Sugar (Pre/Post/Fasting)	Weight	Temp
	__AM __PM	/				__Pre__Post__Fasting		

Symptoms/Notes:

Date	Time	Blood Pressure	Heart Rate	Resp Rate	Oxygen Level	Blood Sugar (Pre/Post/Fasting)	Weight	Temp
	__AM __PM	/				__Pre__Post__Fasting		

Symptoms/Notes:

Date	Time	Blood Pressure	Heart Rate	Resp Rate	Oxygen Level	Blood Sugar (Pre/Post/Fasting)	Weight	Temp
	__AM __PM	/				__Pre__Post__Fasting		

Symptoms/Notes:

Date	Time	Blood Pressure	Heart Rate	Resp Rate	Oxygen Level	Blood Sugar (Pre/Post/Fasting)	Weight	Temp
	__AM __PM	/				__Pre__Post__Fasting		

Symptoms/Notes:

Date	Time	Blood Pressure	Heart Rate	Resp Rate	Oxygen Level	Blood Sugar (Pre/Post/Fasting)	Weight	Temp
	__AM __PM	/				__Pre__Post__Fasting		

Symptoms/Notes:

Date	Time	Blood Pressure	Heart Rate	Resp Rate	Oxygen Level	Blood Sugar (Pre/Post/Fasting)	Weight	Temp
	__AM __PM	/				__Pre__Post__Fasting		

Symptoms/Notes:

Date	Time	Blood Pressure	Heart Rate	Resp Rate	Oxygen Level	Blood Sugar (Pre/Post/Fasting)	Weight	Temp
	__AM __PM	/				__Pre__Post__Fasting		

Symptoms/Notes:

Date	Time	Blood Pressure	Heart Rate	Resp Rate	Oxygen Level	Blood Sugar (Pre/Post/Fasting)	Weight	Temp
	__AM __PM	/				__Pre__Post__Fasting		

Symptoms/Notes:

Date	Time	Blood Pressure	Heart Rate	Resp Rate	Oxygen Level	Blood Sugar (Pre/Post/Fasting)	Weight	Temp
	__AM __PM	/				__Pre__Post__Fasting		

Symptoms/Notes:

Date	Time	Blood Pressure	Heart Rate	Resp Rate	Oxygen Level	Blood Sugar (Pre/Post/Fasting)	Weight	Temp
	__AM __PM	/				__Pre__Post__Fasting		

Symptoms/Notes:

Date	Time	Blood Pressure	Heart Rate	Resp Rate	Oxygen Level	Blood Sugar (Pre/Post/Fasting)	Weight	Temp
	__AM __PM	/				__Pre__Post__Fasting		

Symptoms/Notes:

Date	Time	Blood Pressure	Heart Rate	Resp Rate	Oxygen Level	Blood Sugar (Pre/Post/Fasting)	Weight	Temp
	__AM __PM	/				__Pre__Post__Fasting		

Symptoms/Notes:

Date	Time	Blood Pressure	Heart Rate	Resp Rate	Oxygen Level	Blood Sugar (Pre/Post/Fasting)	Weight	Temp
	__AM __PM	/				__Pre__Post__Fasting		

Symptoms/Notes:

Date	Time	Blood Pressure	Heart Rate	Resp Rate	Oxygen Level	Blood Sugar (Pre/Post/Fasting)	Weight	Temp
	__AM __PM	/				__Pre__Post__Fasting		

Symptoms/Notes:

Date	Time	Blood Pressure	Heart Rate	Resp Rate	Oxygen Level	Blood Sugar (Pre/Post/Fasting)	Weight	Temp
	__AM __PM	/				__Pre__Post__Fasting		

Symptoms/Notes:

Date	Time	Blood Pressure	Heart Rate	Resp Rate	Oxygen Level	Blood Sugar (Pre/Post/Fasting)	Weight	Temp
	__AM __PM	/				__Pre__Post__Fasting		

Symptoms/Notes:

Date	Time	Blood Pressure	Heart Rate	Resp Rate	Oxygen Level	Blood Sugar (Pre/Post/Fasting)	Weight	Temp
	__AM __PM	/				__Pre__Post__Fasting		

Symptoms/Notes:

Date	Time	Blood Pressure	Heart Rate	Resp Rate	Oxygen Level	Blood Sugar (Pre/Post/Fasting)	Weight	Temp
	__AM __PM	/				__Pre__Post__Fasting		

Symptoms/Notes:

Date	Time	Blood Pressure	Heart Rate	Resp Rate	Oxygen Level	Blood Sugar (Pre/Post/Fasting)	Weight	Temp
	__AM __PM	/				__Pre__Post__Fasting		

Symptoms/Notes:

Date	Time	Blood Pressure	Heart Rate	Resp Rate	Oxygen Level	Blood Sugar (Pre/Post/Fasting)	Weight	Temp
	__AM __PM	/				__Pre__Post__Fasting		

Symptoms/Notes:

Date	Time	Blood Pressure	Heart Rate	Resp Rate	Oxygen Level	Blood Sugar (Pre/Post/Fasting)	Weight	Temp
	__AM __PM	/				__Pre__Post__Fasting		

Symptoms/Notes:

Date	Time	Blood Pressure	Heart Rate	Resp Rate	Oxygen Level	Blood Sugar (Pre/Post/Fasting)	Weight	Temp
	__AM __PM	/				__Pre__Post__Fasting		

Symptoms/Notes:

Date	Time	Blood Pressure	Heart Rate	Resp Rate	Oxygen Level	Blood Sugar (Pre/Post/Fasting)	Weight	Temp
	__AM __PM	/				__Pre__Post__Fasting		

Symptoms/Notes:

Date	Time	Blood Pressure	Heart Rate	Resp Rate	Oxygen Level	Blood Sugar (Pre/Post/Fasting)	Weight	Temp
	__AM __PM	/				__Pre__Post__Fasting		

Symptoms/Notes:

Date	Time	Blood Pressure	Heart Rate	Resp Rate	Oxygen Level	Blood Sugar (Pre/Post/Fasting)	Weight	Temp
	__AM __PM	/				__Pre__Post__Fasting		

Symptoms/Notes:

Date	Time	Blood Pressure	Heart Rate	Resp Rate	Oxygen Level	Blood Sugar (Pre/Post/Fasting)	Weight	Temp
	__AM __PM	/				__Pre__Post__Fasting		

Symptoms/Notes:

Date	Time	Blood Pressure	Heart Rate	Resp Rate	Oxygen Level	Blood Sugar (Pre/Post/Fasting)	Weight	Temp
	__AM __PM	/				__Pre__Post__Fasting		

Symptoms/Notes:

Date	Time	Blood Pressure	Heart Rate	Resp Rate	Oxygen Level	Blood Sugar (Pre/Post/Fasting)	Weight	Temp
	__AM __PM	/				__Pre__Post__Fasting		

Symptoms/Notes:

Date	Time	Blood Pressure	Heart Rate	Resp Rate	Oxygen Level	Blood Sugar (Pre/Post/Fasting)	Weight	Temp
	__AM __PM	/				__Pre__Post__Fasting		

Symptoms/Notes:

Date	Time	Blood Pressure	Heart Rate	Resp Rate	Oxygen Level	Blood Sugar (Pre/Post/Fasting)	Weight	Temp
	__AM __PM	/				__Pre__Post__Fasting		

Symptoms/Notes:

Date	Time	Blood Pressure	Heart Rate	Resp Rate	Oxygen Level	Blood Sugar (Pre/Post/Fasting)	Weight	Temp
	__AM __PM	/				__Pre__Post__Fasting		

Symptoms/Notes:

Date	Time	Blood Pressure	Heart Rate	Resp Rate	Oxygen Level	Blood Sugar (Pre/Post/Fasting)	Weight	Temp
	__AM __PM	/				__Pre__Post__Fasting		

Symptoms/Notes:

Date	Time	Blood Pressure	Heart Rate	Resp Rate	Oxygen Level	Blood Sugar (Pre/Post/Fasting)	Weight	Temp
	__AM __PM	/				__Pre__Post__Fasting		

Symptoms/Notes:

Date	Time	Blood Pressure	Heart Rate	Resp Rate	Oxygen Level	Blood Sugar (Pre/Post/Fasting)	Weight	Temp
	__AM __PM	/				__Pre__Post__Fasting		

Symptoms/Notes:

Date	Time	Blood Pressure	Heart Rate	Resp Rate	Oxygen Level	Blood Sugar (Pre/Post/Fasting)	Weight	Temp
	__AM __PM	/				__Pre__Post__Fasting		

Symptoms/Notes:

Date	Time	Blood Pressure	Heart Rate	Resp Rate	Oxygen Level	Blood Sugar (Pre/Post/Fasting)	Weight	Temp
	__AM __PM	/				__Pre__Post__Fasting		

Symptoms/Notes:

Date	Time	Blood Pressure	Heart Rate	Resp Rate	Oxygen Level	Blood Sugar (Pre/Post/Fasting)	Weight	Temp
	__AM __PM	/				__Pre__Post__Fasting		

Symptoms/Notes:

Date	Time	Blood Pressure	Heart Rate	Resp Rate	Oxygen Level	Blood Sugar (Pre/Post/Fasting)	Weight	Temp
	__AM __PM	/				__Pre__Post__Fasting		

Symptoms/Notes:

Date	Time	Blood Pressure	Heart Rate	Resp Rate	Oxygen Level	Blood Sugar (Pre/Post/Fasting)	Weight	Temp
	__AM __PM	/				__Pre__Post__Fasting		

Symptoms/Notes:

Date	Time	Blood Pressure	Heart Rate	Resp Rate	Oxygen Level	Blood Sugar (Pre/Post/Fasting)	Weight	Temp
	__AM __PM	/				__Pre__Post__Fasting		

Symptoms/Notes:

Date	Time	Blood Pressure	Heart Rate	Resp Rate	Oxygen Level	Blood Sugar (Pre/Post/Fasting)	Weight	Temp
	__AM __PM	/				__Pre__Post__Fasting		

Symptoms/Notes:

Date	Time	Blood Pressure	Heart Rate	Resp Rate	Oxygen Level	Blood Sugar (Pre/Post/Fasting)	Weight	Temp
	__AM __PM	/				__Pre__Post__Fasting		

Symptoms/Notes:

Date	Time	Blood Pressure	Heart Rate	Resp Rate	Oxygen Level	Blood Sugar (Pre/Post/Fasting)	Weight	Temp
	__AM __PM	/				__Pre__Post__Fasting		

Symptoms/Notes:

Date	Time	Blood Pressure	Heart Rate	Resp Rate	Oxygen Level	Blood Sugar (Pre/Post/Fasting)	Weight	Temp
	__AM __PM	/				__Pre__Post__Fasting		

Symptoms/Notes:

Date	Time	Blood Pressure	Heart Rate	Resp Rate	Oxygen Level	Blood Sugar (Pre/Post/Fasting)	Weight	Temp
	__AM __PM	/				__Pre__Post__Fasting		

Symptoms/Notes:

Date	Time	Blood Pressure	Heart Rate	Resp Rate	Oxygen Level	Blood Sugar (Pre/Post/Fasting)	Weight	Temp
	__AM __PM	/				__Pre__Post__Fasting		

Symptoms/Notes:

Date	Time	Blood Pressure	Heart Rate	Resp Rate	Oxygen Level	Blood Sugar (Pre/Post/Fasting)	Weight	Temp
	__AM __PM	/				__Pre__Post__Fasting		

Symptoms/Notes:

Date	Time	Blood Pressure	Heart Rate	Resp Rate	Oxygen Level	Blood Sugar (Pre/Post/Fasting)	Weight	Temp
	__AM __PM	/				__Pre__Post__Fasting		

Symptoms/Notes:

Date	Time	Blood Pressure	Heart Rate	Resp Rate	Oxygen Level	Blood Sugar (Pre/Post/Fasting)	Weight	Temp
	__AM __PM	/				__Pre__Post__Fasting		

Symptoms/Notes:

Date	Time	Blood Pressure	Heart Rate	Resp Rate	Oxygen Level	Blood Sugar (Pre/Post/Fasting)	Weight	Temp
	__AM __PM	/				__Pre__Post__Fasting		

Symptoms/Notes:

Date	Time	Blood Pressure	Heart Rate	Resp Rate	Oxygen Level	Blood Sugar (Pre/Post/Fasting)	Weight	Temp
	__AM __PM	/				__Pre__Post__Fasting		

Symptoms/Notes:

Date	Time	Blood Pressure	Heart Rate	Resp Rate	Oxygen Level	Blood Sugar (Pre/Post/Fasting)	Weight	Temp
	__AM __PM	/				__Pre__Post__Fasting		

Symptoms/Notes:

Date	Time	Blood Pressure	Heart Rate	Resp Rate	Oxygen Level	Blood Sugar (Pre/Post/Fasting)	Weight	Temp
	__AM __PM	/				__Pre__Post__Fasting		

Symptoms/Notes:

Date	Time	Blood Pressure	Heart Rate	Resp Rate	Oxygen Level	Blood Sugar (Pre/Post/Fasting)	Weight	Temp
	__AM __PM	/				__Pre__Post__Fasting		

Symptoms/Notes:

Date	Time	Blood Pressure	Heart Rate	Resp Rate	Oxygen Level	Blood Sugar (Pre/Post/Fasting)	Weight	Temp
	__AM __PM	/				__Pre__Post__Fasting		

Symptoms/Notes:

Date	Time	Blood Pressure	Heart Rate	Resp Rate	Oxygen Level	Blood Sugar (Pre/Post/Fasting)	Weight	Temp
	__AM __PM	/				__Pre__Post__Fasting		

Symptoms/Notes:

Date	Time	Blood Pressure	Heart Rate	Resp Rate	Oxygen Level	Blood Sugar (Pre/Post/Fasting)	Weight	Temp
	__AM __PM	/				__Pre__Post__Fasting		

Symptoms/Notes:

Date	Time	Blood Pressure	Heart Rate	Resp Rate	Oxygen Level	Blood Sugar (Pre/Post/Fasting)	Weight	Temp
	__AM __PM	/				__Pre__Post__Fasting		

Symptoms/Notes:

Date	Time	Blood Pressure	Heart Rate	Resp Rate	Oxygen Level	Blood Sugar (Pre/Post/Fasting)	Weight	Temp
	__AM __PM	/				__Pre__Post__Fasting		

Symptoms/Notes:

Date	Time	Blood Pressure	Heart Rate	Resp Rate	Oxygen Level	Blood Sugar (Pre/Post/Fasting)	Weight	Temp
	__AM __PM	/				__Pre__Post__Fasting		

Symptoms/Notes:

Date	Time	Blood Pressure	Heart Rate	Resp Rate	Oxygen Level	Blood Sugar (Pre/Post/Fasting)	Weight	Temp
	__AM __PM	/				__Pre__Post__Fasting		

Symptoms/Notes:

Date	Time	Blood Pressure	Heart Rate	Resp Rate	Oxygen Level	Blood Sugar (Pre/Post/Fasting)	Weight	Temp
	__AM __PM	/				__Pre__Post__Fasting		

Symptoms/Notes:

Date	Time	Blood Pressure	Heart Rate	Resp Rate	Oxygen Level	Blood Sugar (Pre/Post/Fasting)	Weight	Temp
	__AM __PM	/				__Pre__Post__Fasting		

Symptoms/Notes:

Date	Time	Blood Pressure	Heart Rate	Resp Rate	Oxygen Level	Blood Sugar (Pre/Post/Fasting)	Weight	Temp
	__AM __PM	/				__Pre__Post__Fasting		

Symptoms/Notes:

Date	Time	Blood Pressure	Heart Rate	Resp Rate	Oxygen Level	Blood Sugar (Pre/Post/Fasting)	Weight	Temp
	__AM __PM	/				__Pre__Post__Fasting		

Symptoms/Notes:

Date	Time	Blood Pressure	Heart Rate	Resp Rate	Oxygen Level	Blood Sugar (Pre/Post/Fasting)	Weight	Temp
	__AM __PM	/				__Pre__Post__Fasting		

Symptoms/Notes:

Date	Time	Blood Pressure	Heart Rate	Resp Rate	Oxygen Level	Blood Sugar (Pre/Post/Fasting)	Weight	Temp
	__AM __PM	/				__Pre__Post__Fasting		

Symptoms/Notes:

Date	Time	Blood Pressure	Heart Rate	Resp Rate	Oxygen Level	Blood Sugar (Pre/Post/Fasting)	Weight	Temp
	__AM __PM	/				__Pre__Post__Fasting		

Symptoms/Notes:

Date	Time	Blood Pressure	Heart Rate	Resp Rate	Oxygen Level	Blood Sugar (Pre/Post/Fasting)	Weight	Temp
	__AM __PM	/				__Pre__Post__Fasting		

Symptoms/Notes:

Date	Time	Blood Pressure	Heart Rate	Resp Rate	Oxygen Level	Blood Sugar (Pre/Post/Fasting)	Weight	Temp
	__AM __PM	/				__Pre__Post__Fasting		

Symptoms/Notes:

Date	Time	Blood Pressure	Heart Rate	Resp Rate	Oxygen Level	Blood Sugar (Pre/Post/Fasting)	Weight	Temp
	__AM __PM	/				__Pre__Post__Fasting		

Symptoms/Notes:

Date	Time	Blood Pressure	Heart Rate	Resp Rate	Oxygen Level	Blood Sugar (Pre/Post/Fasting)	Weight	Temp
	__AM __PM	/				__Pre__Post__Fasting		

Symptoms/Notes:

Date	Time	Blood Pressure	Heart Rate	Resp Rate	Oxygen Level	Blood Sugar (Pre/Post/Fasting)	Weight	Temp
	__AM __PM	/				__Pre__Post__Fasting		

Symptoms/Notes:

Date	Time	Blood Pressure	Heart Rate	Resp Rate	Oxygen Level	Blood Sugar (Pre/Post/Fasting)	Weight	Temp
	__AM __PM	/				__Pre__Post__Fasting		

Symptoms/Notes:

Date	Time	Blood Pressure	Heart Rate	Resp Rate	Oxygen Level	Blood Sugar (Pre/Post/Fasting)	Weight	Temp
	__AM __PM	/				__Pre__Post__Fasting		

Symptoms/Notes:

Date	Time	Blood Pressure	Heart Rate	Resp Rate	Oxygen Level	Blood Sugar (Pre/Post/Fasting)	Weight	Temp
	__AM __PM	/				__Pre__Post__Fasting		

Symptoms/Notes:

Date	Time	Blood Pressure	Heart Rate	Resp Rate	Oxygen Level	Blood Sugar (Pre/Post/Fasting)	Weight	Temp
	__AM __PM	/				__Pre__Post__Fasting		

Symptoms/Notes:

Date	Time	Blood Pressure	Heart Rate	Resp Rate	Oxygen Level	Blood Sugar (Pre/Post/Fasting)	Weight	Temp
	__AM __PM	/				__Pre__Post__Fasting		

Symptoms/Notes:

Date	Time	Blood Pressure	Heart Rate	Resp Rate	Oxygen Level	Blood Sugar (Pre/Post/Fasting)	Weight	Temp
	__AM __PM	/				__Pre__Post__Fasting		

Symptoms/Notes:

Date	Time	Blood Pressure	Heart Rate	Resp Rate	Oxygen Level	Blood Sugar (Pre/Post/Fasting)	Weight	Temp
	__AM __PM	/				__Pre__Post__Fasting		

Symptoms/Notes:

Date	Time	Blood Pressure	Heart Rate	Resp Rate	Oxygen Level	Blood Sugar (Pre/Post/Fasting)	Weight	Temp
	__AM __PM	/				__Pre__Post__Fasting		

Symptoms/Notes:

Date	Time	Blood Pressure	Heart Rate	Resp Rate	Oxygen Level	Blood Sugar (Pre/Post/Fasting)	Weight	Temp
	__AM __PM	/				__Pre__Post__Fasting		

Symptoms/Notes:

Date	Time	Blood Pressure	Heart Rate	Resp Rate	Oxygen Level	Blood Sugar (Pre/Post/Fasting)	Weight	Temp
	__AM __PM	/				__Pre__Post__Fasting		

Symptoms/Notes:

Date	Time	Blood Pressure	Heart Rate	Resp Rate	Oxygen Level	Blood Sugar (Pre/Post/Fasting)	Weight	Temp
	__AM __PM	/				__Pre__Post__Fasting		

Symptoms/Notes:

Date	Time	Blood Pressure	Heart Rate	Resp Rate	Oxygen Level	Blood Sugar (Pre/Post/Fasting)	Weight	Temp
	__AM __PM	/				__Pre__Post__Fasting		

Symptoms/Notes:

Date	Time	Blood Pressure	Heart Rate	Resp Rate	Oxygen Level	Blood Sugar (Pre/Post/Fasting)	Weight	Temp
	__AM __PM	/				__Pre__Post__Fasting		

Symptoms/Notes:

Date	Time	Blood Pressure	Heart Rate	Resp Rate	Oxygen Level	Blood Sugar (Pre/Post/Fasting)	Weight	Temp
	__AM __PM	/				__Pre__Post__Fasting		

Symptoms/Notes:

Date	Time	Blood Pressure	Heart Rate	Resp Rate	Oxygen Level	Blood Sugar (Pre/Post/Fasting)	Weight	Temp
	__AM __PM	/				__Pre__Post__Fasting		

Symptoms/Notes:

Date	Time	Blood Pressure	Heart Rate	Resp Rate	Oxygen Level	Blood Sugar (Pre/Post/Fasting)	Weight	Temp
	__AM __PM	/				__Pre__Post__Fasting		

Symptoms/Notes:

Date	Time	Blood Pressure	Heart Rate	Resp Rate	Oxygen Level	Blood Sugar (Pre/Post/Fasting)	Weight	Temp
	__AM __PM	/				__Pre__Post__Fasting		

Symptoms/Notes:

Date	Time	Blood Pressure	Heart Rate	Resp Rate	Oxygen Level	Blood Sugar (Pre/Post/Fasting)	Weight	Temp
	__AM __PM	/				__Pre__Post__Fasting		

Symptoms/Notes:

Date	Time	Blood Pressure	Heart Rate	Resp Rate	Oxygen Level	Blood Sugar (Pre/Post/Fasting)	Weight	Temp
	__AM __PM	/				__Pre__Post__Fasting		

Symptoms/Notes:

Date	Time	Blood Pressure	Heart Rate	Resp Rate	Oxygen Level	Blood Sugar (Pre/Post/Fasting)	Weight	Temp
	__AM __PM	/				__Pre__Post__Fasting		

Symptoms/Notes:

Date	Time	Blood Pressure	Heart Rate	Resp Rate	Oxygen Level	Blood Sugar (Pre/Post/Fasting)	Weight	Temp
	__AM __PM	/				__Pre__Post__Fasting		

Symptoms/Notes:

Date	Time	Blood Pressure	Heart Rate	Resp Rate	Oxygen Level	Blood Sugar (Pre/Post/Fasting)	Weight	Temp
	__AM __PM	/				__Pre__Post__Fasting		

Symptoms/Notes:

Date	Time	Blood Pressure	Heart Rate	Resp Rate	Oxygen Level	Blood Sugar (Pre/Post/Fasting)	Weight	Temp
	__AM __PM	/				__Pre__Post__Fasting		

Symptoms/Notes:

Date	Time	Blood Pressure	Heart Rate	Resp Rate	Oxygen Level	Blood Sugar (Pre/Post/Fasting)	Weight	Temp
	__AM __PM	/				__Pre__Post__Fasting		

Symptoms/Notes:

Date	Time	Blood Pressure	Heart Rate	Resp Rate	Oxygen Level	Blood Sugar (Pre/Post/Fasting)	Weight	Temp
	__AM __PM	/				__Pre__Post__Fasting		

Symptoms/Notes:

Date	Time	Blood Pressure	Heart Rate	Resp Rate	Oxygen Level	Blood Sugar (Pre/Post/Fasting)	Weight	Temp
	__AM __PM	/				__Pre__Post__Fasting		

Symptoms/Notes:

Date	Time	Blood Pressure	Heart Rate	Resp Rate	Oxygen Level	Blood Sugar (Pre/Post/Fasting)	Weight	Temp
	__AM __PM	/				__Pre__Post__Fasting		

Symptoms/Notes:

Date	Time	Blood Pressure	Heart Rate	Resp Rate	Oxygen Level	Blood Sugar (Pre/Post/Fasting)	Weight	Temp
	__AM __PM	/				__Pre__Post__Fasting		

Symptoms/Notes:

Date	Time	Blood Pressure	Heart Rate	Resp Rate	Oxygen Level	Blood Sugar (Pre/Post/Fasting)	Weight	Temp
	__AM __PM	/				__Pre__Post__Fasting		

Symptoms/Notes:

Date	Time	Blood Pressure	Heart Rate	Resp Rate	Oxygen Level	Blood Sugar (Pre/Post/Fasting)	Weight	Temp
	__AM __PM	/				__Pre__Post__Fasting		

Symptoms/Notes:

Date	Time	Blood Pressure	Heart Rate	Resp Rate	Oxygen Level	Blood Sugar (Pre/Post/Fasting)	Weight	Temp
	__AM __PM	/				__Pre__Post__Fasting		

Symptoms/Notes:

Date	Time	Blood Pressure	Heart Rate	Resp Rate	Oxygen Level	Blood Sugar (Pre/Post/Fasting)	Weight	Temp
	__AM __PM	/				__Pre__Post__Fasting		

Symptoms/Notes:

Date	Time	Blood Pressure	Heart Rate	Resp Rate	Oxygen Level	Blood Sugar (Pre/Post/Fasting)	Weight	Temp
	__AM __PM	/				__Pre__Post__Fasting		

Symptoms/Notes:

Date	Time	Blood Pressure	Heart Rate	Resp Rate	Oxygen Level	Blood Sugar (Pre/Post/Fasting)	Weight	Temp
	__AM __PM	/				__Pre__Post__Fasting		

Symptoms/Notes:

Date	Time	Blood Pressure	Heart Rate	Resp Rate	Oxygen Level	Blood Sugar (Pre/Post/Fasting)	Weight	Temp
	__AM __PM	/				__Pre__Post__Fasting		

Symptoms/Notes:

Date	Time	Blood Pressure	Heart Rate	Resp Rate	Oxygen Level	Blood Sugar (Pre/Post/Fasting)	Weight	Temp
	__AM __PM	/				__Pre__Post__Fasting		

Symptoms/Notes:

Date	Time	Blood Pressure	Heart Rate	Resp Rate	Oxygen Level	Blood Sugar (Pre/Post/Fasting)	Weight	Temp
	__AM __PM	/				__Pre__Post__Fasting		

Symptoms/Notes:

Date	Time	Blood Pressure	Heart Rate	Resp Rate	Oxygen Level	Blood Sugar (Pre/Post/Fasting)	Weight	Temp
	__AM __PM	/				__Pre__Post__Fasting		

Symptoms/Notes:

Date	Time	Blood Pressure	Heart Rate	Resp Rate	Oxygen Level	Blood Sugar (Pre/Post/Fasting)	Weight	Temp
	__AM __PM	/				__Pre__Post__Fasting		

Symptoms/Notes:

Date	Time	Blood Pressure	Heart Rate	Resp Rate	Oxygen Level	Blood Sugar (Pre/Post/Fasting)	Weight	Temp
	__AM __PM	/				__Pre__Post__Fasting		

Symptoms/Notes:

Date	Time	Blood Pressure	Heart Rate	Resp Rate	Oxygen Level	Blood Sugar (Pre/Post/Fasting)	Weight	Temp
	__AM __PM	/				__Pre__Post__Fasting		

Symptoms/Notes:

Date	Time	Blood Pressure	Heart Rate	Resp Rate	Oxygen Level	Blood Sugar (Pre/Post/Fasting)	Weight	Temp
	__AM __PM	/				__Pre__Post__Fasting		

Symptoms/Notes:

Date	Time	Blood Pressure	Heart Rate	Resp Rate	Oxygen Level	Blood Sugar (Pre/Post/Fasting)	Weight	Temp
	__AM __PM	/				__Pre__Post__Fasting		

Symptoms/Notes:

Date	Time	Blood Pressure	Heart Rate	Resp Rate	Oxygen Level	Blood Sugar (Pre/Post/Fasting)	Weight	Temp
	__AM __PM	/				__Pre__Post__Fasting		

Symptoms/Notes:

Date	Time	Blood Pressure	Heart Rate	Resp Rate	Oxygen Level	Blood Sugar (Pre/Post/Fasting)	Weight	Temp
	__AM __PM	/				__Pre__Post__Fasting		

Symptoms/Notes:

Date	Time	Blood Pressure	Heart Rate	Resp Rate	Oxygen Level	Blood Sugar (Pre/Post/Fasting)	Weight	Temp
	__AM __PM	/				__Pre__Post__Fasting		

Symptoms/Notes:

Date	Time	Blood Pressure	Heart Rate	Resp Rate	Oxygen Level	Blood Sugar (Pre/Post/Fasting)	Weight	Temp
	__AM __PM	/				__Pre__Post__Fasting		

Symptoms/Notes:

Date	Time	Blood Pressure	Heart Rate	Resp Rate	Oxygen Level	Blood Sugar (Pre/Post/Fasting)	Weight	Temp
	__AM __PM	/				__Pre__Post__Fasting		

Symptoms/Notes:

Date	Time	Blood Pressure	Heart Rate	Resp Rate	Oxygen Level	Blood Sugar (Pre/Post/Fasting)	Weight	Temp
	__AM __PM	/				__Pre __Post __Fasting		

Symptoms/Notes:

Date	Time	Blood Pressure	Heart Rate	Resp Rate	Oxygen Level	Blood Sugar (Pre/Post/Fasting)	Weight	Temp
	__AM __PM	/				__Pre __Post __Fasting		

Symptoms/Notes:

Date	Time	Blood Pressure	Heart Rate	Resp Rate	Oxygen Level	Blood Sugar (Pre/Post/Fasting)	Weight	Temp
	__AM __PM	/				__Pre __Post __Fasting		

Symptoms/Notes:

Date	Time	Blood Pressure	Heart Rate	Resp Rate	Oxygen Level	Blood Sugar (Pre/Post/Fasting)	Weight	Temp
	__AM __PM	/				__Pre __Post __Fasting		

Symptoms/Notes:

Date	Time	Blood Pressure	Heart Rate	Resp Rate	Oxygen Level	Blood Sugar (Pre/Post/Fasting)	Weight	Temp
	__AM __PM	/				__Pre __Post __Fasting		

Symptoms/Notes:

Date	Time	Blood Pressure	Heart Rate	Resp Rate	Oxygen Level	Blood Sugar (Pre/Post/Fasting)	Weight	Temp
	__AM __PM	/				__Pre __Post __Fasting		

Symptoms/Notes:

Date	Time	Blood Pressure	Heart Rate	Resp Rate	Oxygen Level	Blood Sugar (Pre/Post/Fasting)	Weight	Temp
	__AM __PM	/				__Pre __Post __Fasting		

Symptoms/Notes:

Date	Time	Blood Pressure	Heart Rate	Resp Rate	Oxygen Level	Blood Sugar (Pre/Post/Fasting)	Weight	Temp
	__AM __PM	/				__Pre__Post__Fasting		

Symptoms/Notes:

Date	Time	Blood Pressure	Heart Rate	Resp Rate	Oxygen Level	Blood Sugar (Pre/Post/Fasting)	Weight	Temp
	__AM __PM	/				__Pre__Post__Fasting		

Symptoms/Notes:

Date	Time	Blood Pressure	Heart Rate	Resp Rate	Oxygen Level	Blood Sugar (Pre/Post/Fasting)	Weight	Temp
	__AM __PM	/				__Pre__Post__Fasting		

Symptoms/Notes:

Date	Time	Blood Pressure	Heart Rate	Resp Rate	Oxygen Level	Blood Sugar (Pre/Post/Fasting)	Weight	Temp
	__AM __PM	/				__Pre__Post__Fasting		

Symptoms/Notes:

Date	Time	Blood Pressure	Heart Rate	Resp Rate	Oxygen Level	Blood Sugar (Pre/Post/Fasting)	Weight	Temp
	__AM __PM	/				__Pre__Post__Fasting		

Symptoms/Notes:

Date	Time	Blood Pressure	Heart Rate	Resp Rate	Oxygen Level	Blood Sugar (Pre/Post/Fasting)	Weight	Temp
	__AM __PM	/				__Pre__Post__Fasting		

Symptoms/Notes:

Date	Time	Blood Pressure	Heart Rate	Resp Rate	Oxygen Level	Blood Sugar (Pre/Post/Fasting)	Weight	Temp
	__AM __PM	/				__Pre__Post__Fasting		

Symptoms/Notes:

Date	Time	Blood Pressure	Heart Rate	Resp Rate	Oxygen Level	Blood Sugar (Pre/Post/Fasting)	Weight	Temp
	__AM __PM	/				__Pre__Post__Fasting		

Symptoms/Notes:

Date	Time	Blood Pressure	Heart Rate	Resp Rate	Oxygen Level	Blood Sugar (Pre/Post/Fasting)	Weight	Temp
	__AM __PM	/				__Pre__Post__Fasting		

Symptoms/Notes:

Date	Time	Blood Pressure	Heart Rate	Resp Rate	Oxygen Level	Blood Sugar (Pre/Post/Fasting)	Weight	Temp
	__AM __PM	/				__Pre__Post__Fasting		

Symptoms/Notes:

Date	Time	Blood Pressure	Heart Rate	Resp Rate	Oxygen Level	Blood Sugar (Pre/Post/Fasting)	Weight	Temp
	__AM __PM	/				__Pre__Post__Fasting		

Symptoms/Notes:

Date	Time	Blood Pressure	Heart Rate	Resp Rate	Oxygen Level	Blood Sugar (Pre/Post/Fasting)	Weight	Temp
	__AM __PM	/				__Pre__Post__Fasting		

Symptoms/Notes:

Date	Time	Blood Pressure	Heart Rate	Resp Rate	Oxygen Level	Blood Sugar (Pre/Post/Fasting)	Weight	Temp
	__AM __PM	/				__Pre__Post__Fasting		

Symptoms/Notes:

Date	Time	Blood Pressure	Heart Rate	Resp Rate	Oxygen Level	Blood Sugar (Pre/Post/Fasting)	Weight	Temp
	__AM __PM	/				__Pre__Post__Fasting		

Symptoms/Notes:

Date	Time	Blood Pressure	Heart Rate	Resp Rate	Oxygen Level	Blood Sugar (Pre/Post/Fasting)	Weight	Temp
	__AM __PM	/				__Pre__Post__Fasting		

Symptoms/Notes:

Date	Time	Blood Pressure	Heart Rate	Resp Rate	Oxygen Level	Blood Sugar (Pre/Post/Fasting)	Weight	Temp
	__AM __PM	/				__Pre__Post__Fasting		

Symptoms/Notes:

Date	Time	Blood Pressure	Heart Rate	Resp Rate	Oxygen Level	Blood Sugar (Pre/Post/Fasting)	Weight	Temp
	__AM __PM	/				__Pre__Post__Fasting		

Symptoms/Notes:

Date	Time	Blood Pressure	Heart Rate	Resp Rate	Oxygen Level	Blood Sugar (Pre/Post/Fasting)	Weight	Temp
	__AM __PM	/				__Pre__Post__Fasting		

Symptoms/Notes:

Date	Time	Blood Pressure	Heart Rate	Resp Rate	Oxygen Level	Blood Sugar (Pre/Post/Fasting)	Weight	Temp
	__AM __PM	/				__Pre__Post__Fasting		

Symptoms/Notes:

Date	Time	Blood Pressure	Heart Rate	Resp Rate	Oxygen Level	Blood Sugar (Pre/Post/Fasting)	Weight	Temp
	__AM __PM	/				__Pre__Post__Fasting		

Symptoms/Notes:

Date	Time	Blood Pressure	Heart Rate	Resp Rate	Oxygen Level	Blood Sugar (Pre/Post/Fasting)	Weight	Temp
	__AM __PM	/				__Pre__Post__Fasting		

Symptoms/Notes:

Date	Time	Blood Pressure	Heart Rate	Resp Rate	Oxygen Level	Blood Sugar (Pre/Post/Fasting)	Weight	Temp
	__AM __PM	/				__Pre__Post__Fasting		

Symptoms/Notes:

Date	Time	Blood Pressure	Heart Rate	Resp Rate	Oxygen Level	Blood Sugar (Pre/Post/Fasting)	Weight	Temp
	__AM __PM	/				__Pre__Post__Fasting		

Symptoms/Notes:

Date	Time	Blood Pressure	Heart Rate	Resp Rate	Oxygen Level	Blood Sugar (Pre/Post/Fasting)	Weight	Temp
	__AM __PM	/				__Pre__Post__Fasting		

Symptoms/Notes:

Date	Time	Blood Pressure	Heart Rate	Resp Rate	Oxygen Level	Blood Sugar (Pre/Post/Fasting)	Weight	Temp
	__AM __PM	/				__Pre__Post__Fasting		

Symptoms/Notes:

Date	Time	Blood Pressure	Heart Rate	Resp Rate	Oxygen Level	Blood Sugar (Pre/Post/Fasting)	Weight	Temp
	__AM __PM	/				__Pre__Post__Fasting		

Symptoms/Notes:

Date	Time	Blood Pressure	Heart Rate	Resp Rate	Oxygen Level	Blood Sugar (Pre/Post/Fasting)	Weight	Temp
	__AM __PM	/				__Pre__Post__Fasting		

Symptoms/Notes:

Date	Time	Blood Pressure	Heart Rate	Resp Rate	Oxygen Level	Blood Sugar (Pre/Post/Fasting)	Weight	Temp
	__AM __PM	/				__Pre__Post__Fasting		

Symptoms/Notes:

Date	Time	Blood Pressure	Heart Rate	Resp Rate	Oxygen Level	Blood Sugar (Pre/Post/Fasting)	Weight	Temp
	__AM __PM	/				__Pre__Post__Fasting		

Symptoms/Notes:

Date	Time	Blood Pressure	Heart Rate	Resp Rate	Oxygen Level	Blood Sugar (Pre/Post/Fasting)	Weight	Temp
	__AM __PM	/				__Pre__Post__Fasting		

Symptoms/Notes:

Date	Time	Blood Pressure	Heart Rate	Resp Rate	Oxygen Level	Blood Sugar (Pre/Post/Fasting)	Weight	Temp
	__AM __PM	/				__Pre__Post__Fasting		

Symptoms/Notes:

Date	Time	Blood Pressure	Heart Rate	Resp Rate	Oxygen Level	Blood Sugar (Pre/Post/Fasting)	Weight	Temp
	__AM __PM	/				__Pre__Post__Fasting		

Symptoms/Notes:

Date	Time	Blood Pressure	Heart Rate	Resp Rate	Oxygen Level	Blood Sugar (Pre/Post/Fasting)	Weight	Temp
	__AM __PM	/				__Pre__Post__Fasting		

Symptoms/Notes:

Date	Time	Blood Pressure	Heart Rate	Resp Rate	Oxygen Level	Blood Sugar (Pre/Post/Fasting)	Weight	Temp
	__AM __PM	/				__Pre__Post__Fasting		

Symptoms/Notes:

Date	Time	Blood Pressure	Heart Rate	Resp Rate	Oxygen Level	Blood Sugar (Pre/Post/Fasting)	Weight	Temp
	__AM __PM	/				__Pre__Post__Fasting		

Symptoms/Notes:

Date	Time	Blood Pressure	Heart Rate	Resp Rate	Oxygen Level	Blood Sugar (Pre/Post/Fasting)	Weight	Temp
	__AM __PM	/				__Pre__Post__Fasting		

Symptoms/Notes:

Date	Time	Blood Pressure	Heart Rate	Resp Rate	Oxygen Level	Blood Sugar (Pre/Post/Fasting)	Weight	Temp
	__AM __PM	/				__Pre__Post__Fasting		

Symptoms/Notes:

Date	Time	Blood Pressure	Heart Rate	Resp Rate	Oxygen Level	Blood Sugar (Pre/Post/Fasting)	Weight	Temp
	__AM __PM	/				__Pre__Post__Fasting		

Symptoms/Notes:

Date	Time	Blood Pressure	Heart Rate	Resp Rate	Oxygen Level	Blood Sugar (Pre/Post/Fasting)	Weight	Temp
	__AM __PM	/				__Pre__Post__Fasting		

Symptoms/Notes:

Date	Time	Blood Pressure	Heart Rate	Resp Rate	Oxygen Level	Blood Sugar (Pre/Post/Fasting)	Weight	Temp
	__AM __PM	/				__Pre__Post__Fasting		

Symptoms/Notes:

Date	Time	Blood Pressure	Heart Rate	Resp Rate	Oxygen Level	Blood Sugar (Pre/Post/Fasting)	Weight	Temp
	__AM __PM	/				__Pre__Post__Fasting		

Symptoms/Notes:

Date	Time	Blood Pressure	Heart Rate	Resp Rate	Oxygen Level	Blood Sugar (Pre/Post/Fasting)	Weight	Temp
	__AM __PM	/				__Pre__Post__Fasting		

Symptoms/Notes:

Date	Time	Blood Pressure	Heart Rate	Resp Rate	Oxygen Level	Blood Sugar (Pre/Post/Fasting)	Weight	Temp
	__AM __PM	/				__Pre__Post__Fasting		

Symptoms/Notes:

Date	Time	Blood Pressure	Heart Rate	Resp Rate	Oxygen Level	Blood Sugar (Pre/Post/Fasting)	Weight	Temp
	__AM __PM	/				__Pre__Post__Fasting		

Symptoms/Notes:

Date	Time	Blood Pressure	Heart Rate	Resp Rate	Oxygen Level	Blood Sugar (Pre/Post/Fasting)	Weight	Temp
	__AM __PM	/				__Pre__Post__Fasting		

Symptoms/Notes:

Date	Time	Blood Pressure	Heart Rate	Resp Rate	Oxygen Level	Blood Sugar (Pre/Post/Fasting)	Weight	Temp
	__AM __PM	/				__Pre__Post__Fasting		

Symptoms/Notes:

Date	Time	Blood Pressure	Heart Rate	Resp Rate	Oxygen Level	Blood Sugar (Pre/Post/Fasting)	Weight	Temp
	__AM __PM	/				__Pre__Post__Fasting		

Symptoms/Notes:

Date	Time	Blood Pressure	Heart Rate	Resp Rate	Oxygen Level	Blood Sugar (Pre/Post/Fasting)	Weight	Temp
	__AM __PM	/				__Pre__Post__Fasting		

Symptoms/Notes:

Date	Time	Blood Pressure	Heart Rate	Resp Rate	Oxygen Level	Blood Sugar (Pre/Post/Fasting)	Weight	Temp
	__AM __PM	/				__Pre__Post__Fasting		

Symptoms/Notes:

Date	Time	Blood Pressure	Heart Rate	Resp Rate	Oxygen Level	Blood Sugar (Pre/Post/Fasting)	Weight	Temp
	__AM __PM	/				__Pre__Post__Fasting		

Symptoms/Notes:

Date	Time	Blood Pressure	Heart Rate	Resp Rate	Oxygen Level	Blood Sugar (Pre/Post/Fasting)	Weight	Temp
	__AM __PM	/				__Pre__Post__Fasting		

Symptoms/Notes:

Date	Time	Blood Pressure	Heart Rate	Resp Rate	Oxygen Level	Blood Sugar (Pre/Post/Fasting)	Weight	Temp
	__AM __PM	/				__Pre__Post__Fasting		

Symptoms/Notes:

Date	Time	Blood Pressure	Heart Rate	Resp Rate	Oxygen Level	Blood Sugar (Pre/Post/Fasting)	Weight	Temp
	__AM __PM	/				__Pre__Post__Fasting		

Symptoms/Notes:

Date	Time	Blood Pressure	Heart Rate	Resp Rate	Oxygen Level	Blood Sugar (Pre/Post/Fasting)	Weight	Temp
	__AM __PM	/				__Pre__Post__Fasting		

Symptoms/Notes:

Date	Time	Blood Pressure	Heart Rate	Resp Rate	Oxygen Level	Blood Sugar (Pre/Post/Fasting)	Weight	Temp
	__AM __PM	/				__Pre__Post__Fasting		

Symptoms/Notes:

Date	Time	Blood Pressure	Heart Rate	Resp Rate	Oxygen Level	Blood Sugar (Pre/Post/Fasting)	Weight	Temp
	__AM __PM	/				__Pre__Post__Fasting		

Symptoms/Notes:

Date	Time	Blood Pressure	Heart Rate	Resp Rate	Oxygen Level	Blood Sugar (Pre/Post/Fasting)	Weight	Temp
	__AM __PM	/				__Pre__Post__Fasting		

Symptoms/Notes:

Date	Time	Blood Pressure	Heart Rate	Resp Rate	Oxygen Level	Blood Sugar (Pre/Post/Fasting)	Weight	Temp
	__AM __PM	/				__Pre__Post__Fasting		

Symptoms/Notes:

Date	Time	Blood Pressure	Heart Rate	Resp Rate	Oxygen Level	Blood Sugar (Pre/Post/Fasting)	Weight	Temp
	__AM __PM	/				__Pre__Post__Fasting		

Symptoms/Notes:

Date	Time	Blood Pressure	Heart Rate	Resp Rate	Oxygen Level	Blood Sugar (Pre/Post/Fasting)	Weight	Temp
	__AM __PM	/				__Pre__Post__Fasting		

Symptoms/Notes:

Date	Time	Blood Pressure	Heart Rate	Resp Rate	Oxygen Level	Blood Sugar (Pre/Post/Fasting)	Weight	Temp
	__AM __PM	/				__Pre__Post__Fasting		

Symptoms/Notes:

Date	Time	Blood Pressure	Heart Rate	Resp Rate	Oxygen Level	Blood Sugar (Pre/Post/Fasting)	Weight	Temp
	__AM __PM	/				__Pre__Post__Fasting		

Symptoms/Notes:

Date	Time	Blood Pressure	Heart Rate	Resp Rate	Oxygen Level	Blood Sugar (Pre/Post/Fasting)	Weight	Temp
	__AM __PM	/				__Pre__Post__Fasting		

Symptoms/Notes:

Date	Time	Blood Pressure	Heart Rate	Resp Rate	Oxygen Level	Blood Sugar (Pre/Post/Fasting)	Weight	Temp
	__AM __PM	/				__Pre__Post__Fasting		

Symptoms/Notes:

Date	Time	Blood Pressure	Heart Rate	Resp Rate	Oxygen Level	Blood Sugar (Pre/Post/Fasting)	Weight	Temp
	__AM __PM	/				__Pre__Post__Fasting		

Symptoms/Notes:

Date	Time	Blood Pressure	Heart Rate	Resp Rate	Oxygen Level	Blood Sugar (Pre/Post/Fasting)	Weight	Temp
	__AM __PM	/				__Pre__Post__Fasting		

Symptoms/Notes:

Date	Time	Blood Pressure	Heart Rate	Resp Rate	Oxygen Level	Blood Sugar (Pre/Post/Fasting)	Weight	Temp
	__AM __PM	/				__Pre__Post__Fasting		

Symptoms/Notes:

Date	Time	Blood Pressure	Heart Rate	Resp Rate	Oxygen Level	Blood Sugar (Pre/Post/Fasting)	Weight	Temp
	__AM __PM	/				__Pre__Post__Fasting		

Symptoms/Notes:

Date	Time	Blood Pressure	Heart Rate	Resp Rate	Oxygen Level	Blood Sugar (Pre/Post/Fasting)	Weight	Temp
	__AM __PM	/				__Pre__Post__Fasting		

Symptoms/Notes:

Date	Time	Blood Pressure	Heart Rate	Resp Rate	Oxygen Level	Blood Sugar (Pre/Post/Fasting)	Weight	Temp
	__AM __PM	/				__Pre__Post__Fasting		

Symptoms/Notes:

Date	Time	Blood Pressure	Heart Rate	Resp Rate	Oxygen Level	Blood Sugar (Pre/Post/Fasting)	Weight	Temp
	__AM __PM	/				__Pre__Post__Fasting		

Symptoms/Notes:

Date	Time	Blood Pressure	Heart Rate	Resp Rate	Oxygen Level	Blood Sugar (Pre/Post/Fasting)	Weight	Temp
	__AM __PM	/				__Pre__Post__Fasting		

Symptoms/Notes:

Date	Time	Blood Pressure	Heart Rate	Resp Rate	Oxygen Level	Blood Sugar (Pre/Post/Fasting)	Weight	Temp
	__AM __PM	/				__Pre__Post__Fasting		

Symptoms/Notes:

Date	Time	Blood Pressure	Heart Rate	Resp Rate	Oxygen Level	Blood Sugar (Pre/Post/Fasting)	Weight	Temp
	__AM __PM	/				__Pre__Post__Fasting		

Symptoms/Notes:

Date	Time	Blood Pressure	Heart Rate	Resp Rate	Oxygen Level	Blood Sugar (Pre/Post/Fasting)	Weight	Temp
	__AM __PM	/				__Pre__Post__Fasting		

Symptoms/Notes:

Date	Time	Blood Pressure	Heart Rate	Resp Rate	Oxygen Level	Blood Sugar (Pre/Post/Fasting)	Weight	Temp
	__AM __PM	/				__Pre__Post__Fasting		

Symptoms/Notes:

Date	Time	Blood Pressure	Heart Rate	Resp Rate	Oxygen Level	Blood Sugar (Pre/Post/Fasting)	Weight	Temp
	__AM __PM	/				__Pre__Post__Fasting		

Symptoms/Notes:

Date	Time	Blood Pressure	Heart Rate	Resp Rate	Oxygen Level	Blood Sugar (Pre/Post/Fasting)	Weight	Temp
	__AM __PM	/				__Pre__Post__Fasting		

Symptoms/Notes:

Date	Time	Blood Pressure	Heart Rate	Resp Rate	Oxygen Level	Blood Sugar (Pre/Post/Fasting)	Weight	Temp
	__AM __PM	/				__Pre__Post__Fasting		

Symptoms/Notes:

Date	Time	Blood Pressure	Heart Rate	Resp Rate	Oxygen Level	Blood Sugar (Pre/Post/Fasting)	Weight	Temp
	__AM __PM	/				__Pre__Post__Fasting		

Symptoms/Notes:

Date	Time	Blood Pressure	Heart Rate	Resp Rate	Oxygen Level	Blood Sugar (Pre/Post/Fasting)	Weight	Temp
	__AM __PM	/				__Pre__Post__Fasting		

Symptoms/Notes:

Date	Time	Blood Pressure	Heart Rate	Resp Rate	Oxygen Level	Blood Sugar (Pre/Post/Fasting)	Weight	Temp
	__AM __PM	/				__Pre__Post__Fasting		

Symptoms/Notes:

Date	Time	Blood Pressure	Heart Rate	Resp Rate	Oxygen Level	Blood Sugar (Pre/Post/Fasting)	Weight	Temp
	__AM __PM	/				__Pre__Post__Fasting		

Symptoms/Notes:

Date	Time	Blood Pressure	Heart Rate	Resp Rate	Oxygen Level	Blood Sugar (Pre/Post/Fasting)	Weight	Temp
	__AM __PM	/				__Pre__Post__Fasting		

Symptoms/Notes:

Date	Time	Blood Pressure	Heart Rate	Resp Rate	Oxygen Level	Blood Sugar (Pre/Post/Fasting)	Weight	Temp
	__AM __PM	/				__Pre__Post__Fasting		

Symptoms/Notes:

Date	Time	Blood Pressure	Heart Rate	Resp Rate	Oxygen Level	Blood Sugar (Pre/Post/Fasting)	Weight	Temp
	__AM __PM	/				__Pre__Post__Fasting		

Symptoms/Notes:

Date	Time	Blood Pressure	Heart Rate	Resp Rate	Oxygen Level	Blood Sugar (Pre/Post/Fasting)	Weight	Temp
	__AM __PM	/				__Pre__Post__Fasting		

Symptoms/Notes:

Date	Time	Blood Pressure	Heart Rate	Resp Rate	Oxygen Level	Blood Sugar (Pre/Post/Fasting)	Weight	Temp
	__AM __PM	/				__Pre__Post__Fasting		

Symptoms/Notes:

Date	Time	Blood Pressure	Heart Rate	Resp Rate	Oxygen Level	Blood Sugar (Pre/Post/Fasting)	Weight	Temp
	__AM __PM	/				__Pre__Post__Fasting		

Symptoms/Notes:

Date	Time	Blood Pressure	Heart Rate	Resp Rate	Oxygen Level	Blood Sugar (Pre/Post/Fasting)	Weight	Temp
	__AM __PM	/				__Pre__Post__Fasting		

Symptoms/Notes:

Date	Time	Blood Pressure	Heart Rate	Resp Rate	Oxygen Level	Blood Sugar (Pre/Post/Fasting)	Weight	Temp
	__AM __PM	/				__Pre__Post__Fasting		

Symptoms/Notes:

Date	Time	Blood Pressure	Heart Rate	Resp Rate	Oxygen Level	Blood Sugar (Pre/Post/Fasting)	Weight	Temp
	__AM __PM	/				__Pre__Post__Fasting		

Symptoms/Notes:

Date	Time	Blood Pressure	Heart Rate	Resp Rate	Oxygen Level	Blood Sugar (Pre/Post/Fasting)	Weight	Temp
	__AM __PM	/				__Pre__Post__Fasting		

Symptoms/Notes:

Date	Time	Blood Pressure	Heart Rate	Resp Rate	Oxygen Level	Blood Sugar (Pre/Post/Fasting)	Weight	Temp
	__AM __PM	/				__Pre__Post__Fasting		

Symptoms/Notes:

Date	Time	Blood Pressure	Heart Rate	Resp Rate	Oxygen Level	Blood Sugar (Pre/Post/Fasting)	Weight	Temp
	__AM __PM	/				__Pre__Post__Fasting		

Symptoms/Notes:

Date	Time	Blood Pressure	Heart Rate	Resp Rate	Oxygen Level	Blood Sugar (Pre/Post/Fasting)	Weight	Temp
	__AM __PM	/				__Pre__Post__Fasting		

Symptoms/Notes:

Date	Time	Blood Pressure	Heart Rate	Resp Rate	Oxygen Level	Blood Sugar (Pre/Post/Fasting)	Weight	Temp
	__AM __PM	/				__Pre__Post__Fasting		

Symptoms/Notes:

Date	Time	Blood Pressure	Heart Rate	Resp Rate	Oxygen Level	Blood Sugar (Pre/Post/Fasting)	Weight	Temp
	__AM __PM	/				__Pre__Post__Fasting		

Symptoms/Notes:

Date	Time	Blood Pressure	Heart Rate	Resp Rate	Oxygen Level	Blood Sugar (Pre/Post/Fasting)	Weight	Temp
	__AM __PM	/				__Pre__Post__Fasting		

Symptoms/Notes:

Date	Time	Blood Pressure	Heart Rate	Resp Rate	Oxygen Level	Blood Sugar (Pre/Post/Fasting)	Weight	Temp
	__AM __PM	/				__Pre__Post__Fasting		

Symptoms/Notes:

Date	Time	Blood Pressure	Heart Rate	Resp Rate	Oxygen Level	Blood Sugar (Pre/Post/Fasting)	Weight	Temp
	__AM __PM	/				__Pre__Post__Fasting		

Symptoms/Notes:

Date	Time	Blood Pressure	Heart Rate	Resp Rate	Oxygen Level	Blood Sugar (Pre/Post/Fasting)	Weight	Temp
	__AM __PM	/				__Pre__Post__Fasting		

Symptoms/Notes:

Date	Time	Blood Pressure	Heart Rate	Resp Rate	Oxygen Level	Blood Sugar (Pre/Post/Fasting)	Weight	Temp
	__AM __PM	/				__Pre__Post__Fasting		

Symptoms/Notes:

Date	Time	Blood Pressure	Heart Rate	Resp Rate	Oxygen Level	Blood Sugar (Pre/Post/Fasting)	Weight	Temp
	__AM __PM	/				__Pre__Post__Fasting		

Symptoms/Notes:

Date	Time	Blood Pressure	Heart Rate	Resp Rate	Oxygen Level	Blood Sugar (Pre/Post/Fasting)	Weight	Temp
	__AM __PM	/				__Pre__Post__Fasting		

Symptoms/Notes:

Date	Time	Blood Pressure	Heart Rate	Resp Rate	Oxygen Level	Blood Sugar (Pre/Post/Fasting)	Weight	Temp
	__AM __PM	/				__Pre__Post__Fasting		

Symptoms/Notes:

Date	Time	Blood Pressure	Heart Rate	Resp Rate	Oxygen Level	Blood Sugar (Pre/Post/Fasting)	Weight	Temp
	__AM __PM	/				__Pre__Post__Fasting		

Symptoms/Notes:

Date	Time	Blood Pressure	Heart Rate	Resp Rate	Oxygen Level	Blood Sugar (Pre/Post/Fasting)	Weight	Temp
	__AM __PM	/				__Pre__Post__Fasting		

Symptoms/Notes:

Date	Time	Blood Pressure	Heart Rate	Resp Rate	Oxygen Level	Blood Sugar (Pre/Post/Fasting)	Weight	Temp
	__AM __PM	/				__Pre__Post__Fasting		

Symptoms/Notes:

Date	Time	Blood Pressure	Heart Rate	Resp Rate	Oxygen Level	Blood Sugar (Pre/Post/Fasting)	Weight	Temp
	__AM __PM	/				__Pre__Post__Fasting		

Symptoms/Notes:

Date	Time	Blood Pressure	Heart Rate	Resp Rate	Oxygen Level	Blood Sugar (Pre/Post/Fasting)	Weight	Temp
	__AM __PM	/				__Pre__Post__Fasting		

Symptoms/Notes:

Date	Time	Blood Pressure	Heart Rate	Resp Rate	Oxygen Level	Blood Sugar (Pre/Post/Fasting)	Weight	Temp
	__AM __PM	/				__Pre__Post__Fasting		

Symptoms/Notes:

Date	Time	Blood Pressure	Heart Rate	Resp Rate	Oxygen Level	Blood Sugar (Pre/Post/Fasting)	Weight	Temp
	__AM __PM	/				__Pre__Post__Fasting		

Symptoms/Notes:

Date	Time	Blood Pressure	Heart Rate	Resp Rate	Oxygen Level	Blood Sugar (Pre/Post/Fasting)	Weight	Temp
	__AM __PM	/				__Pre__Post__Fasting		

Symptoms/Notes:

Date	Time	Blood Pressure	Heart Rate	Resp Rate	Oxygen Level	Blood Sugar (Pre/Post/Fasting)	Weight	Temp
	__AM __PM	/				__Pre__Post__Fasting		

Symptoms/Notes:

Date	Time	Blood Pressure	Heart Rate	Resp Rate	Oxygen Level	Blood Sugar (Pre/Post/Fasting)	Weight	Temp
	__AM __PM	/				__Pre__Post__Fasting		

Symptoms/Notes:

Date	Time	Blood Pressure	Heart Rate	Resp Rate	Oxygen Level	Blood Sugar (Pre/Post/Fasting)	Weight	Temp
	__AM __PM	/				__Pre__Post__Fasting		

Symptoms/Notes:

Date	Time	Blood Pressure	Heart Rate	Resp Rate	Oxygen Level	Blood Sugar (Pre/Post/Fasting)	Weight	Temp
	__AM __PM	/				__Pre__Post__Fasting		

Symptoms/Notes:

Date	Time	Blood Pressure	Heart Rate	Resp Rate	Oxygen Level	Blood Sugar (Pre/Post/Fasting)	Weight	Temp
	__AM __PM	/				__Pre__Post__Fasting		

Symptoms/Notes:

Date	Time	Blood Pressure	Heart Rate	Resp Rate	Oxygen Level	Blood Sugar (Pre/Post/Fasting)	Weight	Temp
	__AM __PM	/				__Pre__Post__Fasting		

Symptoms/Notes:

Date	Time	Blood Pressure	Heart Rate	Resp Rate	Oxygen Level	Blood Sugar (Pre/Post/Fasting)	Weight	Temp
	__AM __PM	/				__Pre__Post__Fasting		

Symptoms/Notes:

Date	Time	Blood Pressure	Heart Rate	Resp Rate	Oxygen Level	Blood Sugar (Pre/Post/Fasting)	Weight	Temp
	__AM __PM	/				__Pre__Post__Fasting		

Symptoms/Notes:

Date	Time	Blood Pressure	Heart Rate	Resp Rate	Oxygen Level	Blood Sugar (Pre/Post/Fasting)	Weight	Temp
	__AM __PM	/				__Pre__Post__Fasting		

Symptoms/Notes:

Date	Time	Blood Pressure	Heart Rate	Resp Rate	Oxygen Level	Blood Sugar (Pre/Post/Fasting)	Weight	Temp
	__AM __PM	/				__Pre__Post__Fasting		

Symptoms/Notes:

Date	Time	Blood Pressure	Heart Rate	Resp Rate	Oxygen Level	Blood Sugar (Pre/Post/Fasting)	Weight	Temp
	__AM __PM	/				__Pre__Post__Fasting		

Symptoms/Notes:

Date	Time	Blood Pressure	Heart Rate	Resp Rate	Oxygen Level	Blood Sugar (Pre/Post/Fasting)	Weight	Temp
	__AM __PM	/				__Pre__Post__Fasting		

Symptoms/Notes:

Date	Time	Blood Pressure	Heart Rate	Resp Rate	Oxygen Level	Blood Sugar (Pre/Post/Fasting)	Weight	Temp
	__AM __PM	/				__Pre__Post__Fasting		

Symptoms/Notes:

Date	Time	Blood Pressure	Heart Rate	Resp Rate	Oxygen Level	Blood Sugar (Pre/Post/Fasting)	Weight	Temp
	__AM __PM	/				__Pre__Post__Fasting		

Symptoms/Notes:

Date	Time	Blood Pressure	Heart Rate	Resp Rate	Oxygen Level	Blood Sugar (Pre/Post/Fasting)	Weight	Temp
	__AM __PM	/				__Pre__Post__Fasting		

Symptoms/Notes:

Date	Time	Blood Pressure	Heart Rate	Resp Rate	Oxygen Level	Blood Sugar (Pre/Post/Fasting)	Weight	Temp
	__AM __PM	/				__Pre__Post__Fasting		

Symptoms/Notes:

Date	Time	Blood Pressure	Heart Rate	Resp Rate	Oxygen Level	Blood Sugar (Pre/Post/Fasting)	Weight	Temp
	__AM __PM	/				__Pre__Post__Fasting		

Symptoms/Notes:

Date	Time	Blood Pressure	Heart Rate	Resp Rate	Oxygen Level	Blood Sugar (Pre/Post/Fasting)	Weight	Temp
	__AM __PM	/				__Pre__Post__Fasting		

Symptoms/Notes:

Date	Time	Blood Pressure	Heart Rate	Resp Rate	Oxygen Level	Blood Sugar (Pre/Post/Fasting)	Weight	Temp
	__AM __PM	/				__Pre__Post__Fasting		

Symptoms/Notes:

Date	Time	Blood Pressure	Heart Rate	Resp Rate	Oxygen Level	Blood Sugar (Pre/Post/Fasting)	Weight	Temp
	__AM __PM	/				__Pre__Post__Fasting		

Symptoms/Notes:

Date	Time	Blood Pressure	Heart Rate	Resp Rate	Oxygen Level	Blood Sugar (Pre/Post/Fasting)	Weight	Temp
	__AM __PM	/				__Pre__Post__Fasting		

Symptoms/Notes:

Date	Time	Blood Pressure	Heart Rate	Resp Rate	Oxygen Level	Blood Sugar (Pre/Post/Fasting)	Weight	Temp
	__AM __PM	/				__Pre__Post__Fasting		

Symptoms/Notes:

Date	Time	Blood Pressure	Heart Rate	Resp Rate	Oxygen Level	Blood Sugar (Pre/Post/Fasting)	Weight	Temp
	__AM __PM	/				__Pre__Post__Fasting		

Symptoms/Notes:

Date	Time	Blood Pressure	Heart Rate	Resp Rate	Oxygen Level	Blood Sugar (Pre/Post/Fasting)	Weight	Temp
	__AM __PM	/				__Pre__Post__Fasting		

Symptoms/Notes:

Date	Time	Blood Pressure	Heart Rate	Resp Rate	Oxygen Level	Blood Sugar (Pre/Post/Fasting)	Weight	Temp
	__AM __PM	/				__Pre__Post__Fasting		

Symptoms/Notes:

Date	Time	Blood Pressure	Heart Rate	Resp Rate	Oxygen Level	Blood Sugar (Pre/Post/Fasting)	Weight	Temp
	__AM __PM	/				__Pre__Post__Fasting		

Symptoms/Notes:

Date	Time	Blood Pressure	Heart Rate	Resp Rate	Oxygen Level	Blood Sugar (Pre/Post/Fasting)	Weight	Temp
	__AM __PM	/				__Pre__Post__Fasting		

Symptoms/Notes:

Date	Time	Blood Pressure	Heart Rate	Resp Rate	Oxygen Level	Blood Sugar (Pre/Post/Fasting)	Weight	Temp
	__AM __PM	/				__Pre__Post__Fasting		

Symptoms/Notes:

Date	Time	Blood Pressure	Heart Rate	Resp Rate	Oxygen Level	Blood Sugar (Pre/Post/Fasting)	Weight	Temp
	__AM __PM	/				__Pre__Post__Fasting		

Symptoms/Notes:

Date	Time	Blood Pressure	Heart Rate	Resp Rate	Oxygen Level	Blood Sugar (Pre/Post/Fasting)	Weight	Temp
	__AM __PM	/				__Pre__Post__Fasting		

Symptoms/Notes:

Date	Time	Blood Pressure	Heart Rate	Resp Rate	Oxygen Level	Blood Sugar (Pre/Post/Fasting)	Weight	Temp
	__AM __PM	/				__Pre__Post__Fasting		

Symptoms/Notes:

Date	Time	Blood Pressure	Heart Rate	Resp Rate	Oxygen Level	Blood Sugar (Pre/Post/Fasting)	Weight	Temp
	__AM __PM	/				__Pre__Post__Fasting		

Symptoms/Notes:

Date	Time	Blood Pressure	Heart Rate	Resp Rate	Oxygen Level	Blood Sugar (Pre/Post/Fasting)	Weight	Temp
	__AM __PM	/				__Pre__Post__Fasting		

Symptoms/Notes:

Date	Time	Blood Pressure	Heart Rate	Resp Rate	Oxygen Level	Blood Sugar (Pre/Post/Fasting)	Weight	Temp
	__AM __PM	/				__Pre__Post__Fasting		

Symptoms/Notes:

Date	Time	Blood Pressure	Heart Rate	Resp Rate	Oxygen Level	Blood Sugar (Pre/Post/Fasting)	Weight	Temp
	__AM __PM	/				__Pre__Post__Fasting		

Symptoms/Notes:

Date	Time	Blood Pressure	Heart Rate	Resp Rate	Oxygen Level	Blood Sugar (Pre/Post/Fasting)	Weight	Temp
	__AM __PM	/				__Pre__Post__Fasting		

Symptoms/Notes:

Date	Time	Blood Pressure	Heart Rate	Resp Rate	Oxygen Level	Blood Sugar (Pre/Post/Fasting)	Weight	Temp
	__AM __PM	/				__Pre__Post__Fasting		

Symptoms/Notes:

Date	Time	Blood Pressure	Heart Rate	Resp Rate	Oxygen Level	Blood Sugar (Pre/Post/Fasting)	Weight	Temp
	__AM __PM	/				__Pre__Post__Fasting		

Symptoms/Notes:

Date	Time	Blood Pressure	Heart Rate	Resp Rate	Oxygen Level	Blood Sugar (Pre/Post/Fasting)	Weight	Temp
	__AM __PM	/				__Pre__Post__Fasting		

Symptoms/Notes:

Date	Time	Blood Pressure	Heart Rate	Resp Rate	Oxygen Level	Blood Sugar (Pre/Post/Fasting)	Weight	Temp
	__AM __PM	/				__Pre__Post__Fasting		

Symptoms/Notes:

Date	Time	Blood Pressure	Heart Rate	Resp Rate	Oxygen Level	Blood Sugar (Pre/Post/Fasting)	Weight	Temp
	__AM __PM	/				__Pre__Post__Fasting		

Symptoms/Notes:

Date	Time	Blood Pressure	Heart Rate	Resp Rate	Oxygen Level	Blood Sugar (Pre/Post/Fasting)	Weight	Temp
	__AM __PM	/				__Pre__Post__Fasting		

Symptoms/Notes:

Date	Time	Blood Pressure	Heart Rate	Resp Rate	Oxygen Level	Blood Sugar (Pre/Post/Fasting)	Weight	Temp
	__AM __PM	/				__Pre__Post__Fasting		

Symptoms/Notes:

Date	Time	Blood Pressure	Heart Rate	Resp Rate	Oxygen Level	Blood Sugar (Pre/Post/Fasting)	Weight	Temp
	__AM __PM	/				__Pre__Post__Fasting		

Symptoms/Notes:

Date	Time	Blood Pressure	Heart Rate	Resp Rate	Oxygen Level	Blood Sugar (Pre/Post/Fasting)	Weight	Temp
	__AM __PM	/				__Pre__Post__Fasting		

Symptoms/Notes:

Date	Time	Blood Pressure	Heart Rate	Resp Rate	Oxygen Level	Blood Sugar (Pre/Post/Fasting)	Weight	Temp
	__AM __PM	/				__Pre__Post__Fasting		

Symptoms/Notes:

Date	Time	Blood Pressure	Heart Rate	Resp Rate	Oxygen Level	Blood Sugar (Pre/Post/Fasting)	Weight	Temp
	__AM __PM	/				__Pre__Post__Fasting		

Symptoms/Notes:

Date	Time	Blood Pressure	Heart Rate	Resp Rate	Oxygen Level	Blood Sugar (Pre/Post/Fasting)	Weight	Temp
	__AM __PM	/				__Pre __Post __Fasting		

Symptoms/Notes:

Date	Time	Blood Pressure	Heart Rate	Resp Rate	Oxygen Level	Blood Sugar (Pre/Post/Fasting)	Weight	Temp
	__AM __PM	/				__Pre __Post __Fasting		

Symptoms/Notes:

Date	Time	Blood Pressure	Heart Rate	Resp Rate	Oxygen Level	Blood Sugar (Pre/Post/Fasting)	Weight	Temp
	__AM __PM	/				__Pre __Post __Fasting		

Symptoms/Notes:

Date	Time	Blood Pressure	Heart Rate	Resp Rate	Oxygen Level	Blood Sugar (Pre/Post/Fasting)	Weight	Temp
	__AM __PM	/				__Pre __Post __Fasting		

Symptoms/Notes:

Date	Time	Blood Pressure	Heart Rate	Resp Rate	Oxygen Level	Blood Sugar (Pre/Post/Fasting)	Weight	Temp
	__AM __PM	/				__Pre __Post __Fasting		

Symptoms/Notes:

Date	Time	Blood Pressure	Heart Rate	Resp Rate	Oxygen Level	Blood Sugar (Pre/Post/Fasting)	Weight	Temp
	__AM __PM	/				__Pre __Post __Fasting		

Symptoms/Notes:

Date	Time	Blood Pressure	Heart Rate	Resp Rate	Oxygen Level	Blood Sugar (Pre/Post/Fasting)	Weight	Temp
	__AM __PM	/				__Pre __Post __Fasting		

Symptoms/Notes:

Date	Time	Blood Pressure	Heart Rate	Resp Rate	Oxygen Level	Blood Sugar (Pre/Post/Fasting)	Weight	Temp
	__AM __PM	/				__Pre__Post__Fasting		

Symptoms/Notes:

Date	Time	Blood Pressure	Heart Rate	Resp Rate	Oxygen Level	Blood Sugar (Pre/Post/Fasting)	Weight	Temp
	__AM __PM	/				__Pre__Post__Fasting		

Symptoms/Notes:

Date	Time	Blood Pressure	Heart Rate	Resp Rate	Oxygen Level	Blood Sugar (Pre/Post/Fasting)	Weight	Temp
	__AM __PM	/				__Pre__Post__Fasting		

Symptoms/Notes:

Date	Time	Blood Pressure	Heart Rate	Resp Rate	Oxygen Level	Blood Sugar (Pre/Post/Fasting)	Weight	Temp
	__AM __PM	/				__Pre__Post__Fasting		

Symptoms/Notes:

Date	Time	Blood Pressure	Heart Rate	Resp Rate	Oxygen Level	Blood Sugar (Pre/Post/Fasting)	Weight	Temp
	__AM __PM	/				__Pre__Post__Fasting		

Symptoms/Notes:

Date	Time	Blood Pressure	Heart Rate	Resp Rate	Oxygen Level	Blood Sugar (Pre/Post/Fasting)	Weight	Temp
	__AM __PM	/				__Pre__Post__Fasting		

Symptoms/Notes:

Date	Time	Blood Pressure	Heart Rate	Resp Rate	Oxygen Level	Blood Sugar (Pre/Post/Fasting)	Weight	Temp
	__AM __PM	/				__Pre__Post__Fasting		

Symptoms/Notes:

Notes

Your feedback is greatly appreciated!

Your feedback, support, and reviews make it possible for us to create high-quality books and serve more people.

It only takes 60 seconds to leave an honest review. Share your feedback and thoughts so others can see the quality of this book.

Find the location where you purchased the book and leave a review. Select a rating and write a couple of sentences.

That's it! Thank you so much for your support.

Review this product

Share your thoughts with other customers

Write a customer review

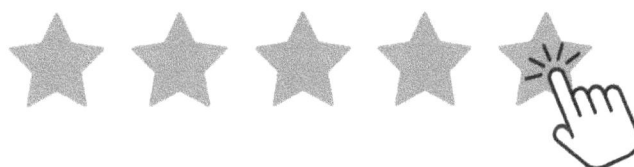

www.ingramcontent.com/pod-product-compliance
Lightning Source LLC
Chambersburg PA
CBHW080422030426
42335CB00020B/2543